OPEN MINDS

A New Perspective on Healing

Rudi Verspoor, FHCH, HD(RHom) DMH

Leonard Levine, MD, DPH, CCFP, DAc

Farid Shodjaee, BSc, DDS

Mary Rothschild, MSW, DHHP, HD(RHom)

James Emmett, BSc, DAc, MMSc, DC

Edited by Serena Williamson, PhD

First Edition

 Book Coach Press

Open Minds
A New Perspective on Healing

Published by:
Book Coach Press
Ottawa, Ontario, Canada
www.BookCoachPress.com
info@BookCoachPress.com

Rudi Verspoor: www.homeopathy.com
Leonard Levine: l.levine@cyberus.ca
Farid Shodjaee: www.drfarid.com
Mary Rothschild: natrldoc@rogers.com
James Emmett: DrEmmett@bellnet.ca
Serena Williamson: www.BookCoachPress.com

Printed in Canada

National Library of Canada Cataloguing in Publication

Open minds : a new perspective on healing / Rudi Verspoor ... [et al.] ; edited by Serena Williamson.

Includes bibliographical references.
ISBN 0-9735207-2-8

1. Alternative medicine. 2. Medical personnel – Attitudes.
I. Verspoor, Rudi, 1950- II. Williamson, Serena, 1948-

R733.O64 2004   615.5   C2004-902822-7

ONLY A BEGINNING

Open Minds is not a medical textbook. The purpose of this publication is to share with you the journeys of traditional western health practitioners who opened their eyes, hearts and minds to additional treatment modalities that they could learn and do with their patients and clients.

The advice in this book is not meant to be a stand-alone replacement for treatments that you or your loved ones may currently be experiencing.

If you are interested in and find yourself moved to explore the various ideas and methods discussed in this book, please contact the authors of the chapters that interest you. They will be happy to meet with you and discuss the various treatment options available to you. They will guide you on your own personal healing journey.

Contents

Introduction

A Fly on the Wall

By Serena Williamson, PhD

The Book Coach
Founder and President, Book Coach Press

About Serena Williamson

Dr. Serena Williamson, The Book Coach and creator of Book Coach Press, works with people who want to write a book, guiding them from inspiration to publication. She helps people get their ideas clear, down onto paper, and out into the world where they belong.

Dr. Serena has counselled people battling cancer, provided advice and direction to a national team of corporate counsellors and taught courses on communication and leadership.

Serena is the author of *Surviving Organizational Insanity: Keeping Spirit Alive at Work; Two Voices/Circle of Love*; the chapter "Write that Book!" in *Expert Women Who Speak: Speak Out*, vol. 3; and *Write That Book! Get it Clear, Get it Down, Get it Out*. Her speaking topics include: Communication Skills; Influencing Skills; Write that Book; and Add Professional Speaking to your Toolkit. Serena has a PhD in Adult Education from the University of Toronto and was the 2003 President of the Ottawa chapter of CAPS, the Canadian Association of Professional Speakers.

Dr. Serena Williamson can be reached at:
www.bookcoachpress.com
info@bookcoachpress.com
613-746-3334

A FLY ON THE WALL

We had just moved to Ottawa in November 1990 when I cracked a tooth. An old molar that was more mercury than enamel had finally given up the battle for survival.

"Dentist, dentist, dentist," I mumbled, flipping the Yellow Pages then scanning the names and numbers to find a practitioner in my area. Relieved to get an appointment quickly, I made my way to the St. Laurent Shopping Centre, discovered the office in the centre's lower level that I hadn't known existed, gave my name to the receptionist, and found myself face-to-face for the first time with Dr. Farid Shodjaee.

What struck me about Farid Shodjaee was his energy, joy and sheer lightness of being. His bright smile and enthusiasm were indescribably contagious. Can a person actually be enthusiastic at the dentist? What impressed me even more about him was his passion and devotion to his craft. My three daughters and I have been his patients all these years and we are ever increasingly impressed with how he is always on the leading edge of his field, going to seminars, conferences and workshops all over the world and constantly presenting us with new discoveries. Farid Shodjaee absolutely loves what he does and inspires confidence in all who are lucky enough to have him for their dentist.

In 1998, my youngest daughter and I moved to California for a year and stayed for three, but we came home twice a year for our dentistry. We could find no one in San Francisco to compare with the treatment and service we received here. Not that we didn't try, we went through two dentists and then gave up.

When we returned to Canada, I was applying for life insurance and needed a medical, but while I had returned to Ottawa, my family doctor had left. Since I loved the way my dentist practised, I thought, why not ask him for a referral? His reply shocked me. "I haven't seen an *allopath* in seven years. Neither has any member of my family." (He has a wife and three sons.)

My quizzical look told him that I had no clue what he was talking about. "We use *homeopathic* medicine," he said emphatically, leading me to believe that *allopath* must mean *non-homeopath*, or regular medical doctor to the rest of the world, like me. He went on to talk about timeline therapy, and how our diseases are anchored in our life events, including various traumas such as a surgery, a broken bone, a marriage break-up or things as seemingly harmless as starting school, getting report cards, or receiving a polio vaccination. He recommended that I see Rudy Verspoor or his wife Patty Smith-Verspoor at their clinic, the Hahnemann Center for Heilkunst.

I stalled, preferring to experience a few more life traumas before I bought Dr. Shodjaee's theories. But I couldn't get it of my mind how happy and healthy he always seemed. Finally, after one more stressful life event, I decided to give Heilkunst a try and called Patty. I quickly became fascinated and began treatment. Simple homeopathic droplets began to change my life.

As I was healing, tight spots showed themselves in my body, places where I was holding tension that needed to be released. Patty recommended James Emmett, the chiropractor, and another new world opened up to me. When James did a chiropractic adjustment, I could feel relaxation spreading throughout my entire body. I could actually experience the energy flowing. I had never had regular chiropractic therapy before and had never even been inclined to try it. Even though my dad raved about chiropractic for his occasional stiff neck, the chiropractor's swift, jarring movements frightened me. The kind of chiropractic that James Emmett practised was a whole other world. In addition, there was something resonant about Farid, Patty and James, as if, even though you were with different practitioners, you were really with the same one in some ways. It began to feel a little spooky. There was a oneness there. Enter Mary Rothschild.

Struggling with a difficult family situation, I called Patty at home for advice. Recognizing that I was on the verge of a powerful breakthrough, Patty recommended that I speak with a psychotherapist. I resisted, she insisted and another exceptional, life-enhancing relationship began. A fabulous, eclectic delightful spirit, Mary Rothschild, opened doors for me and invited me to walk where I had feared to walk before, and there was that resonance again.

Meanwhile, while I visited each of these practitioners, we would spend some time talking about the books they would "one day" write. Now I was becoming the healer. As *The Book Coach* and founder of *Book Coach Press*, I specialize in helping people write that book sooner rather than later. But none of them, with their very busy practices, thought they had the time to write. "One day," they said … I have heard that before. But their resonance intrigued me. I really wanted to be part of those books, *one day*.

Then, *one day*, after a chiropractic treatment, James told me that they were all getting together for a meeting. Boy, did I ever want to be a fly on the wall. I wanted to find out more about how each of them thought, their attitudes toward health and healing, and how they worked together. But I was not a health practitioner. I used to be in the counselling business, but not any more. Now I was a book writing coach. Then it hit me! If I want to be at a meeting of these minds, why couldn't I *create* the meeting, on my terms? Yes!

If these people all wanted to write books but did not have the time, perhaps they would each write a chapter. Bingo! I asked them and they enthusiastically agreed. We had my longed-for meeting at Patty and Rudi's home and the book was born.

Because Rudi Verspoor, Patty's husband and co-founder of the Hahnemann Center for Heilkunst has vast experience writing and is renowned the world over in his field, all authors agreed that Rudi would write the opening and closing chapters, explain homeopathy and Heilkunst and tie the book together.

So why were we doing this book anyway? What was the unifying thread? At first we thought it would be homeopathy, but no. We wanted to open up your medical world. What does the average person know about medicine? They know what their doctor tells them and what they see on television. We are learning more about natural medicine, but who can get a handle on it all? I wanted to share with you my fascination with what I had discovered. I had found a community of medical practitioners who work together to help people heal themselves. In addition, they are each devoted, committed and on the leading edge in their fields.

The book concept seemed great, but something was bothering me. There was one piece missing. We had a dentist, a chiropractor, a psychotherapist and a Homeopath/Heilkunst expert. I wanted a traditional medical doctor, an MD. You see, the whole point of this book was to introduce you to a group of traditional medical practitioners who have undergone healing journeys of their own, discovered new techniques and are offering these to the people they see in their offices. A family physician, a medical doctor, Len Levine completed the picture when I bumped into him at the Heilkunst Center. Although he is now semi-retired, Dr. Levine, already a member of the "spook" group kindly agreed to be part of our book team.

Throughout this project, I have been the coach, encouraging and guiding the authors, editing drafts, badgering them about deadlines and working with our editor, graphic designer, copyeditor and printer to get the book done. It has been a joy working with these people, and an indication to me, and I hope to you too, that if we want something badly enough we can make it happen.

I wanted to work with this team. I also wanted to show you what they have taught me, so that you can see that there is more to healing than pumping ourselves full of medicine. Health happens from the inside out. There is a joy, glow, happiness and a lightness of spirit that is available to all of us. Come let us guide you. See how these doctors' open minds led them to a new perspective on healing.

Chapter One

A Road Map
Finding Your Way Through the Maze

By Rudi Verspoor, FHCH, HD(RHom) DMH

Dean, Hahnemann College for Heilkunst
Director, Hahnemann Center for Heilkunst
Trustee, Hahnemann Center for Heilkunst Trust

About Rudi Verspoor

Rudi Verspoor has been studying Hahnemann's medical system for more than two decades and has acquired extensive clinical experience, particularly relating to complex and chronic cases, in the application of this system. His ongoing research has led to the development of a systematic dynamic approach to therapeutics that is now being offered in a comprehensive form to others through a five-year program.

Rudi Verspoor has written several books and has lectured widely in Canada, the US, the UK and Europe. He served as the Director of the British Institute of Homeopathy Canada from 1993 to 2001, and developed their Homeopathic Practitioner Diploma Program. He helped to found the National United Professional Association of Trained Homeopaths (NUPATH) and the Canadian/International Heilkunst Association (C/IHA). Part of his time is spent advising the Canadian government on health-care policy and in working for greater acceptance of and access to homeopathy and Heilkunst amongst policy makers and the public.

His publications include: *Homeopathy Renewed, A Sequential Approach to the Treatment of Chronic Illness* (with Patty Smith); *A Time for Healing; Homeopathy Re-examined: Beyond the Classical Paradigm* (with Steven Decker); *The Dynamic Legacy: Hahnemann from Homeopathy to Heilkunst* (with Steven Decker). He also has written various articles for Canadian and International journals.

Rudi Verspoor can be reached at:
The Hahnemann College for Heilkunst
2411 River Road, Ottawa ON K4M 1B4
613-692-6950.

A ROAD MAP
FINDING YOUR WAY THROUGH THE MAZE

W hen it comes to understanding the origins of disease, we are pretty much in the dark. Either we are suffering from some "virus," which often remains mysterious and for which there is not much that can be done, or we are given a "diagnosis" in the form of some disease name, and then are prescribed one or more drugs to control the symptoms.

Research money guarantees the search for ever-elusive cures, but when it comes to treatment, the name of the game is always suppression of symptoms. Someone once aptly termed the health-care system a "disease-management system." So, the blood pressure pills control the blood pressure (though not always), and the stomach pills control the acid reflux (though not always), and the painkillers control the migraines (though not always), and you have to keep yourself medicated or the problems return.

For those of you with a thyroid problem or asthma, you must take medication all your life, or so you are told. And although you are grateful for relief, you will likely suffer from side effects, which may or may not be worse than your original symptoms. Eventually you realize that all that is happening is that your symptoms are being suppressed, but the original cause of these symptoms remains. It seems that conventional medicine is good at getting rid of the evidence, but more in the manner of sweeping it under the carpet rather than out the door.

This comes with a huge price tag. Iatrogenic disease (that means disease caused by doctors themselves) is the third-leading cause of death in North America, after cancer and respiratory conditions. And death caused by infections contracted in hospitals is the fourth-leading cause of death.

All in all, despite the impressive technology and the flashy designer drugs, not only is there no real cure going on, you stand a good chance of either being made sicker by conventional medicine, or being killed by it. Some people eventually wake up to the medical merry-go-round that threatens to harm them, and want to get off. They may want off, but don't know how to get off, and stay on only because they think there is no other choice. But there absolutely is a choice!

When you have stepped off that merry-go-round of conventional medicine, you face a bewildering number of therapies and products, each promising to make you well and giving testimonials of cured cases. How can they all promise to fix your ailment? How do you know which one to choose?

The so-called natural health field is a bit of a minefield. Just because something is natural doesn't ensure it is safe or even effective. Lead is natural, but we don't allow it in our gasoline anymore. Mercury is natural, but we don't want it in our teeth. Arsenic is natural, but we know it can kill.

The natural health field talks about supporting our natural healing power, and is generally against intervention, saying, "Let the body do what it was designed to do, it can heal itself, and all we have to do is support that healing." There are many successes with this approach, but also failures.

I treated one woman who had taken many herbs and vitamins, changed her diet and meditated, and found that her symptoms of depression, allergies and chronic fatigue went away, only to return a few years later. The same measures that worked for her before no longer worked, and she wanted to know why.

I remember another young lady with Crohn's Disease (advanced stage of ulcerative colitis) who had recovered under natural therapies, only to see her condition return, worse then ever, after a year. The same therapies, or other natural treatments, no longer worked. She wanted to know why.

I too have wanted to know why. And my search for answers led me to Heilkunst, a logical, rational, scientific system of medicine.

WHAT IS HEILKUNST?

Heilkunst is a little known, yet powerful, system of remediation based on natural law and scientific principles. The term in German comes from two words: heil, which has the dual meaning of cure and healing and kunst, which means the art and science. Thus, at a very simple level it has the basic meaning of "the medical art," but in its deepest sense it means applying the rational approach to making people whole human beings, at all levels – body, mind, soul and spirit. The term "heil" comes from the same root as the Anglo-Saxon "hale" and "hearty."

Heilkunst seeks to remove disease using natural law, and then to restore balance, so that our innate life force can be used for the higher, spiritual purposes of our existence on earth.

MY STORY

My own story is a model of what is wrong with both the conventional medical and natural health fields, and how Heilkunst can provide a better way for the restoration of health consistently, and on clear principles. I think I was your average kid. I got the usual cuts and scrapes. I had the usual round of childhood illnesses of that time – measles, mumps, chicken pox and scarlet fever. I also had my share of tonsillitis and sinusitis. I did perhaps spend more time in the hospital than some. Eventually my tonsils and adenoids were removed and I underwent two hernia operations. I had a lot of dental work, including extraction of my wisdom teeth. I came to hate the smell of antiseptics.

My parents were reasonably typical of that time. When you got sick, you went to bed, drank lots of water and ate a nourishing homemade vegetable or beef and barley broth. While growing up, my family's diet was mostly fresh foods from our garden or homemade canned foods in the winter that we had put away. My parents knew that good health depended on a good foundation. We only took drugs when absolutely necessary, and I can't really remember taking aspirin or antibiotics, except perhaps a few times. My parents didn't like using pesticides and herbicides, and used them as infrequently as possible. We only went to see the doctor when things were serious, or rather, the doctor came to see us!

From a young age, I remember the smell of the hospital, and that old disinfectant they used everywhere. I still vividly recall the horrible pink medicine my mom used to give us when we had pinworms from playing in the neighbouring farms. (Or, rather, *tried* to give us, as we would run and hide when we knew she was coming. Better the pinworms than to have to taste that indescribably awful pink liquid.) This was my introduction to the possibility that the cure might be worse than the disease!

I remember once lying in bed with acute stomach cramps, so severe that my mom finally called the doctor. He came in and tried many things, but nothing worked. I was delirious and just wanted to die. Then he came back, offering me an ugly brown medicine from an old clear glass bottle, which he said would do the trick. I was desperate, so took it. Almost instantly my cramps disappeared and I was flooded with a sense of relief and calm. I asked him what it was, this miracle potion. He told me it was an old formula that he had gotten from a native healer on the Indian Reserve outside of town. It had come from various native plants. This was the first time it occurred to me that there was medicine other than chemical drugs, and that even worked better than they did.

Once I tried to hide in the bathroom when the public health nurse came around to give us the required (or so we thought) vaccinations. I didn't like the thought of a needle, and the shots always made me feel worse for a time after having them. Sometimes I missed them, sometimes they got me on the second pass to round up the stragglers. You win some, lose some, I reasoned at the time. Luckily, there weren't too many vaccinations in my day!

By the time I became a teenager my health seemed quite good. Things were generally fine in university, except for the odd headache, and life overall seemed pretty comfortable. I went abroad after university and had to take a series of special vaccinations (or so they told me). The vaccinations for typhoid, cholera and yellow fever made me feel rundown.

I contracted malaria despite the anti-malarial drugs I had been given to take daily (I later learned they only suppressed the fever, but didn't really protect against malaria, and had side-effects, like blindness.) The tropical disease specialists told me there was nothing to get rid of the malarial parasite. They gave me an experimental drug anyway, and it made me feel as if I was disconnected from reality and walking three feet off the ground. I stopped it after one pill. Better to live with the malaria, I thought!

A dentist told me that I had poor teeth and would likely lose them all by the time I was 40. She didn't tell me what I could do to prevent it other than flossing and brushing, which I had been doing already, with little effect. Then I got married and had children. I had always wanted children and I had an interesting job. Life seemed wonderful and promising, except that I was starting to feel a lack of energy, was getting more frequent sinus headaches, suffering with digestive problems and going through one or two colds and flu every winter. I even started to suffer bouts of depression in the winter months. And my teeth kept getting worse, with serious gum problems and abscesses.

At first I tried to tough it out, but eventually I was driven by my pain and discomfort to see a doctor. I had learned to avoid dentists except in emergencies, as they had no solutions short of surgery. The doctor ran various tests and they all came back negative. He told me nothing was wrong, that I just needed a vacation because I was too stressed (which was true, but vacations were just a temporary relief, like an aspirin for a headache).

The symptoms of my ill health continued and worsened. I went back to the doctors, more in desperation than with any real expectation of help at this point. All sorts of theories were formulated, but in the end they had to admit they didn't have any idea what was going on with me. My illness didn't show up on their radar screen, it had no name, and wasn't "official." I couldn't be given antibiotics, there wasn't a vaccination for me, and it was not yet the age of mass prescription of anti-depressants (luckily for me, I now realize!). I was reluctant to take drugs to begin with, and it particularly bothered me that I was feeling so lousy, yet no one in the medical system knew what was causing it or what to do. I felt like a stateless person, traveling from country to country being rejected by each in turn as I had no nationality or citizenship.

I've always had an inquiring mind. I've always wanted to know the why and how of things. Life is not bearable to me without meaning. And now I wanted to know why I was feeling so sick, even though nothing showed up in the tests and nothing could supposedly be done. In desperation, I went back to what my parents had taught me – to eat fresh foods and to stay away from processed foods with added chemicals. My dad had often said that if you couldn't recognize an ingredient or couldn't pronounce it, it probably wasn't good for you. Nature had given us what we needed. Why did we think we could improve on this?

I remembered the huge vegetable garden that took up our whole back yard and the hours spent working in it, and started my own. I also read books on nutrition, and found a lot of confusion. The experts differed in what was good for you and what wasn't. I felt a little better, and I certainly enjoyed my garden, but underneath my overall condition was getting worse. It took a lot of effort to eat well, or even to know what that meant in the face of all the conflicting opinions, and to take the array of supplements recommended (again, with a lot of conflicting advice). To just keep my head above water seemed to be a full-time job. I began to wonder if there was any light at the end of the tunnel.

I continued to ask doctors for the answers, but without any real sense of hope. I didn't know where else to turn. However, one day I remembered my mother mentioning a "homeopathic" doctor they had had in Holland while I was growing up. I knew the word, even knew how to spell it, but I didn't know what it meant. I went to the local public library and found one book. It opened a door to another world, with a whole different approach to medicine I never even knew existed, but which was the second most popular system of medicine in the world.

I eventually found some local classes on homeopathy and started a natural health program at a local privately-run school. I learned a lot about nutrition, alternative and complementary therapies and diagnostic methods, such as reflexology, acupuncture, shiatsu, massage, iridology, Reiki and yoga.

I learned ways to help my teeth, the ones that were supposed to fall out by the time I was 40. I learned about the problems of mercury toxicity from fillings, of which I had many. I learned that you could do things to improve your vision and get rid of your glasses. My eyes were so bad that I had to now wear glasses to read, and for driving. I started to improve somewhat, but a deeper sense of health still eluded me.

What bothered me just as much as my persistent ill-health was that I had many questions going in, but that I had found few, if any, answers to them coming out of the process. Worse, I came away from my natural health training with even more questions than I had started with. I knew deep down that the answer lay somewhere in the thicket of natural health, so I kept moving forward with my exploration. There was something that drew me in strongly despite my growing frustration. I also knew that the key lay in homeopathy.

Because there were no courses in Canada at the time, I studied with a British school. The more I learned, the more intrigued I became, yet I was still frustrated. Again, I had lots of questions, but no satisfying answers from my teachers. I was told that was the way it was, and was given vague, confusing, or even conflicting answers. Eventually I became a homeopathic physician and started to practise. I had good success, but was still unhappy about what I was doing and the results for my patients. In my questioning I ran up against a mindset that was just as closed, confused and based on authority rather than principle as that of the prevailing system of medicine (which we call allopathy). It was called "classical homeopathy."

I knew there *had* to be more. One day, I was looking for a book to read on a flight home from Europe. I went to the medical section in the hopes there was a book on homeopathy, since homeopathy was much better known in Europe. One book, written in French by a Swiss homeopath, caught my eye. It seemed interesting, promising a different perspective from my classical training.

Well, it not only delivered on its promise, it eventually opened the door to the rational Western medical system I had been looking for all my conscious life, through all my ill-health and suffering. I still vividly recall devouring that book from cover to cover and feeling a sense of elation. I even forgot to eat on the nine-hour flight! I knew I had found the key to unlock the medical system and to make sense of disease, illness and treatment. I just didn't know how to use it.

Then, in my struggles, I met a remarkable guide in the person of Steven Decker, a genius who had been studying a system of health and thought he termed the "Dynamic System." He showed me how classical homeopathy was barring the gate to the full system of medicine developed by the founder of homeopathy, Dr. Samuel Hahnemann, more than 200 years ago. He called it, "allopathy tricked up in chicken feathers." He also showed me that homeopathy was only one part of this amazing system of medicine, called Heilkunst.

After many years of clinical experience and working with Steven, I have been able to put many of the pieces together. If you have ever wondered, as I have, why people get sick, why some get well and others don't, why some things work for one person and not for another, and why, despite doing everything you are supposed to, you are still unwell, and how you decide from the myriad of approaches out there, which is best for you, or what really works, then the explanation that follows is for you.

DISEASE VERSUS IMBALANCE

The foundation to all understanding is in using precise terminology. We toss words around like confetti, and think one is just a synonym for another, including words like sick, ill, disease or imbalance. When you are not feeling well, words aren't that important, you just want to feel better. But words are critical, even vital, to being able to successfully treat. To be sick and to be ill are two different things. All sick people are ill, but not all ill people are sick. And disease and illness are different.

Let me explain. We have a living force within us, a dynamic power that animates us, digests our lunch, keeps us healthy, allows us to think and allows us to grow, learn, change and create. This living force or power, which is called the *Dynamis*, has two aspects, almost like Siamese twins. All cultures and traditions have a term for this living, dynamic power – chi, prana, etc. What is not often realized or emphasized is the *dual nature* of our life force.

One side of the Dynamis simply tries to maintain a state of health, and that is its only job. It has a one-track mind. When you lose your health, it goes to work to restore balance. We call this the *sustentive power* of the Dynamis, as it sustains us in health.

The other side of the Dynamis allows our cells to divide, allows us to generate something new – an idea, a child, a work of art. We call this the *generative power* of the Dynamis, for obvious reasons.

Why is this distinction important? For one thing, it allows us to understand the vital distinction between simply being ill and being sick. Being ill means that you are out of balance. When this power is off balance, you feel ill and not at all well. Your sense of well-being is off. Your normal functions and processes are not working properly because you have an excess, or lack of, something, or too much of something in one part of the body and not enough in another. Say you don't get enough Vitamin C in your food. You start to feel a little tired or your eyes become bloodshot. You simply need to take some Vitamin C and the sustentive power is able to restore balance – the problem is solved. Simple, yet elegant. When you get too hot, you simply have to cool off to feel better. This is known as the law of opposites. It's a natural law, and unlike human law, it doesn't change. There is no disease, just an imbalance in your normal homeostasis which means "balance."

Disease is quite a different matter. Disease is when some external agent or event affects (impinges upon) our generative power. This can be a toxin, a drug, an emotional shock, or an accident such as a concussion. Instead of simply creating an imbalance, these events in some way damage the generative power. This damage, or impingement, is a bit like getting pregnant. No amount of exercise, good food, supplements or rest is going to remove the fact that you are pregnant. You need somehow to reverse the process like reverse time-lapse photography. How can this be done?

That takes us to another reason to understand the dual nature of the Dynamis, our living principle. We saw that the sustentive power is able to restore balance in the case of imbalance when we use the natural law of opposites. But if we have damage to the generative side of the Dynamis, this doesn't work. It can make us feel better; it can strengthen our energy and constitution, but it can't remove the damage. This requires the use of a remedy that is applied according to another natural law – the law of similars.

If you get irritated eyes from cutting onions, you can get rid of this irritation by taking a very small dose of specially prepared onion (*Allium cepa*). Let's say you touch some poison ivy and get a rash with intense itching – using the Law of Similars you can simply take a small dose of poison ivy. This even works preventatively. The pioneers, busy clearing the land and always at risk of poison ivy, learned to make a tea in the spring from the young leaves and to drink it. The tea protected them from reacting to the poison ivy all season. This is an application of the law of similars.

But the law of similars goes beyond this. If someone has a complaint of vomiting and diarrhea, a need for fresh air, but is freezing despite being piled under the covers and in great fear and anxiety, this presents a picture of arsenic poisoning. The person swears, reasonably enough, that they have not ingested any arsenic, but it sure looks like it (it's similar, we say). We would say it's an "arsenic-like disease." So, by the law of similars, I am justified in giving him an energized, diluted dose of arsenic. I'll explain later how this can be done with no risk.

I recall one dramatic case of a woman who called me at 3:00 a.m. from Mexico City with a sudden case of Montezuma's Revenge. She had continual diarrhea and vomiting and was worried. Luckily she had an emergency homeopathic kit with her. I told her to dissolve a few pellets of *Arsenicum album* 30C in some water and to sip on this every few minutes until the symptoms abated and went back to sleep. She told me later, on her return, that she had felt better within minutes and within an hour the symptoms had stopped. In the morning she was almost fully recovered, needing only to drink some extra fluids and restore her lost electrolytes (law of opposites). She called it a miracle, but I called it a simple case of following natural law. Miracles are only good things we experience that we can't explain.

Now we can understand another important distinction, that difference between the disease itself and your body's efforts to *get rid* of disease. This means that disease has two sides: the initial action of the disease agent that dynamically affects the generative power and the counteraction of the sustentive power of the Dynamis.

Let's take a simple case of an infectious disease, like chicken pox. Your child goes to a friend's house and a few days later the mother calls and says that her child has broken out with the characteristic eruptions of chicken pox. Well, we all know that the neighbour's child was infectious for a week to ten days prior to the rash. So now you can expect that your child will come down with the visible symptoms of chicken pox within a week or so. That means that your child already has the disease, which means that your generative power is already infected by the chicken pox microbe. Yet, your child doesn't have any symptoms at this point. These come later. Why?

Remember the sustentive power, the one whose job it is to keep you in health? It starts to make preparations to repel the invader. First, it has to marshal its resources, get its lines of communication clear and prepare the various parts of the immune system to do battle. Then it goes into action. It's this reaction of the sustentive power to the disease itself that produces the characteristic fever, followed by the itching and rash, as well as a general feeling of lassitude, that we suffer and call the disease. It's part of the whole disease process, but not the disease properly speaking.

CHRONIC DISEASE AND HEALING REACTIONS

Why is this important to know, you might ask? Well, it becomes important when we look at the process of cure and healing (remediation) in the case of chronic disease.

Up until now we have used examples of simple disease cases, but what if it's not so simple? Chicken pox will go away on its own eventually, even if you don't do anything, so it is one of the self-limiting diseases. Diseases that don't go away on their own, however, are called chronic diseases. These continue, inexorably, until you die, unless they are cured. They require careful identification so that they can be destroyed. When the right remedy is given on the basis of the law of similars, the disease is *destroyed*, not simply suppressed. This is a very gentle action.

The sustentive power of the Dynamis then is roused to react to the curative action of the medicine. This counter action, called the healing reaction, involves a number of general symptoms such as changes in temperature, mood swings, disturbances of sleep and various discharge reactions at the physical level (nausea, mucous, perspiration, etc.). This *healing reaction* is not always pleasant, but is followed by a general feeling of increased well-being and soundness, as well as an improvement in the disease symptoms the patient was initially complaining about.

I remember one patient who went to bed one night thinking half-seriously she was going to die and waking the next morning feeling great, with a significant removal of her many chronic complaints. This is common with the healing reaction – a period of discomfort is followed by an increased sense of well-being and greater soundness. A critical part of the training of a Heilkunst practitioner (Heilkünstler) is the ability to distinguish the important healing reaction from the counter-action of a disease process.

The problem is that conventional allopathic doctors are trained to see all symptoms as a disease process. The healing reaction is like a house renovation.

There may appear to be a greater mess taking place, but you are not concerned because you can understand and "see" that the house will be greatly improved by the process.

Let's imagine that you come from a planet where people don't renovate their homes. They just let them run down and then build new ones. They also suffer from vandals who attack the weakened homes. You come to earth to visit and see people tearing apart a roof, or taking out old windows. You can only assume that they are vandalizing the house. When your friend explains that they are doing all this to make the house better, you have no frame of reference to understand this.

This is the situation a doctor is in. He has no reference to understand the healing reaction. To him it is only a disease process, and then he uses antipathic (law of opposites) measures to suppress the symptoms of the healing reaction (anti-inflammatories, antibiotics, anti-depressants, etc.) because he has no cure. But this is like pouring water on someone trying to light a fire to burn off refuse. Why? The body's way of healing is to generate an inflammatory process, which marshals the resources of the immune and repair systems to a particular spot. This produces some pain and discomfort, like a home renovation, but then eventually results in a greater level of health and functioning. Antibiotics and anti-inflammatories, for example, act to shut down this process.

INTERNAL AND EXTERNAL BUGS

Despite its technical complexity, conventional medicine is still based on the simplistic premise of Louis Pasteur that the body is aseptic (has no microbes) and that any microbe found has to have come from outside – an unwanted invader. The search for the cause of disease is still the search for a bacteria or virus of some sort. It's true that some diseases are caused by infectious external microbes, but there are many diseases that have no microbial cause.

While conventional medicine latched on to the rather simple notion that each microbial form is unique, other researchers argued, with convincing evidence, that a microbe could alter form under the right conditions. This is termed the polymorphic view, from the Greek term "many forms." What they discovered was that the body itself would produce many different microbial forms when it was stressed. The more stressed it was, the more the body would produce viral and fungal forms, as opposed to bacterial forms. These microbes were not the *cause* of any disease, but rather the *result*.

Supporters of the polymorphic view placed the emphasis of treatment on the underlying state of health of the body, stressing nutrition, hygiene and lifestyle. Further research also showed that bacteria were produced as part of the body's healing reaction; they are the necessary scavengers of the dead tissue that is then replaced with healthy tissue. The use of antibiotics (literally "anti-life" agents) served only to shut down the inflammation and to kill off these beneficial bacteria.

The debate raged in the last part of the 19th and early 20th century between Pasteur's view and that of his colleague, Antoine Bechamp, as to the origin of disease. The Pasteurian view was too rigid. Bechamp's view made allowance for infectious diseases, but also recognized that not all bacterial or viral evidence could be taken as the cause of disease. However, the advent of the patented drug age in the 1940s virtually removed any emphasis in conventional medicine on nutrition and lifestyle, and all treatment focused on finding a drug to kill the presumed bacteria or virus.

Essentially, conventional medicine now assumes that any inflammation is an attempt to fight off a microbial invasion and that any microbe found in the body came from outside and is a disease agent. Ostensibly, in order to be objective, conventional medicine must prove three things (called Koch's postulates) before it can term a microbe a cause of disease rather than just a result of a stressed organism: it must be able to isolate the microbe, culture it outside the body and then inject it into a healthy subject (animal) and cause the disease in each case. The problem is that these conditions are seldom fulfilled, as in the case of the so-called Human Immuno-deficiency Virus (HIV), the supposed cause of AIDS (Acquired Immuno-deficiency Syndrome), or the recent SARS (Sudden Acute Respiratory Syndrome). The virus is not found in all people suffering from these conditions (note they are termed "syndromes") and it is found in only small quantities where it is. It has not been found to cause the disease condition in all cases.

Yet, so strong is the mind-set that the virus found must be a cause, that the strict requirements of Koch's postulates are often ignored or loosely applied and the virus, which is really caused within the body under stress, often from pollution, processed food and chemical drugs, is claimed as the cause. Since viruses are very difficult to treat because they change so rapidly, strong (and costly) drugs are developed to try to control (suppress) the symptoms. These drugs further weaken the immune system, thus causing a negative spiral of ill-health.

WHAT IS DISEASE?

How do we know what is a disease and how do we identify (diagnose) a particular disease when it happens? Earlier, I stated that disease was not simply an imbalance. Disease produces "dis-ease," but it is more than that. It is a form of impregnation of your generative power by a foreign influence that can only be removed (cured) by the use of medicines according to the law of similars.

What we find in conventional medicine is largely the description of an arbitrary condition based on the visible, on physical evidence caused by the counteraction of the sustentive power, not the real diagnosis of the underlying disease. The tip-off these days is that most new "diseases" are termed syndromes, for example Chronic Fatigue Syndrome. Let me illustrate what I mean.

Let's say a doctor finds people who have the same physical symptom, such as painful swelling of the joints. He takes this particular symptom or sign and gives it a name, drawing from Latin or Greek by tradition, and calls it "arthritis." This also gives it some semblance of authority or reality it might not have on its own – arthritis just means inflammation of the joints, which sounds better than simply saying you have inflammation of the joints. The problem is that they have never been able to find the true cause of arthritis. There are lots of theories, but not one cause. That's because arthritis is a condition that is produced in people *by* disease! And each case might have a different disease or series of diseases that caused that particular case of arthritis. In one case, it might be inherited, in another it might be due to chemical exposure, in another it may be deep or prolonged emotional shock.

And in some cases, it might have nothing to do with disease, but is instead caused by poor diet and nutrition (then you need to use the law of opposites – better diet and nutrition!)

The whole world, whether conventional or alternative/complementary, seems to run on these arbitrary conditions. Name any product out there, or any therapy or treatment modality, and you will find cases of seemingly miraculous cures of arthritis from just using a particular product or therapy. Yet, you will find ten cases not helped for every one helped. How can this be? Because of the failure to understand what disease really is.

Imagine we have ten people suffering from stomach (peptic) ulcers, a painful condition if you've ever had one. They are all told first to simply drink more water (75% of people are chronically dehydrated and stomach ulcers is one result). After a few days, one person has a dramatic and immediate recovery. The others notice no or only a slight improvement. Then the remaining nine are told to eat a special diet. Two drop out of the program, cured. Next, we go to some form of energy balancing like acupuncture, shiatsu or Reiki, or exercise to relieve stress and tone the body – another two people leave, happy.

The others are growing frustrated as they see little or no improvement compared to their lucky counterparts. Why don't they get better, they ask? Well, their cause has not been addressed yet. So far, we have been looking at imbalances. Next, we look to see if there is any identifiable disease, such as an emotional shock, a physical trauma, or some inherited factor that has to be addressed with medicine based on the law of similars. One person has had the ulcer since losing his wife or his job. Another has been on other drugs, one of the side-effects being a stomach ulcer from overacidity. A third has had the ulcer after eating contaminated meat or fish while on a trip abroad. Each of these is addressed specifically and they, too, can leave the group. Eventually, all are treated, but using different treatments and for different periods of time depending on the circumstances of their case.

WHAT CAN PRODUCE DISEASE?

- toxins (chemicals, drugs, pollution, vaccinations)

- physical traumas (concussions, broken bones, deep wounds, injections)

- emotional shocks (suppressed grief, fear, shame, anger, etc.)

- infectious microbes (cholera, flu, typhoid, tuberculosis, etc.)

- inherited diseases (more on this later)

- false beliefs about the world (illusions, delusions) – again, more about this later as it requires some explanation.

If you have any of these, they can potentially produce, on their own or in combination, almost any condition imaginable. Conventional medicine simply looks at the visible results, picks the most common symptom and gives it a name, presuming thereby to have identified a disease. If there is any treatment, it is designed really to manage the symptoms, because there can be no true cure for an arbitrary condition.

I remember the case of the woman who came to see me for her daughter's urinary incontinence. I asked her what the conventional diagnosis had been. She said "exercise-induced incontinence." Apparently they hadn't found a Latin or Greek name for this yet! I asked what they had suggested as treatment. She told me, "Nothing." I asked the young teen what sports she played or did. She gave me a long list. I asked her if this happened during all the activities, and she answered no, that it only happened during karate.

I laughed and suggested that they had got the diagnosis wrong. It should have been "karate-induced incontinence!" On further questioning, it turned out that she felt unfairly dealt with by her instructor and had a degree of suppressed anger. I gave her the medicine to deal with suppressed anger and the problem went away.

In another case, a woman came into my office in tears because the doctors had told her that she would have to learn to live with her chronic arthritic pain. She could take aspirin (which didn't really help and caused stomach problems) or move to a dry climate, or suffer. Needless to say, she didn't like any of the options she was offered by the rheumatologist despite the many years of study and impressive degrees behind his name. I told her in all seriousness that we had no cure for arthritis, but that we could remove (cure) the diseases causing it. We were eventually able to remove her arthritic condition, though it took some time due to the many diseases involved.

Heilkunst is a system of medicine that gives you a true identification (diagnosis) of disease, because as soon as you have identified the disease, the curative remedy is automatically known — it is disclosive, not just descriptive. Or, in some cases, where the remedy is known, through the symptoms alone, the nature of the disease is then known. The art lies in the skill of diagnosis, and there are many ways to make this relatively easy to do.

TWO TYPES OF DISEASE

The founder of Heilkunst, Dr. Samuel Hahnemann, discovered that there are two types of disease: diseases that are constant in nature and diseases that are variable. The constant diseases, which we call tonic diseases, are those that always show up in the same manner, such as measles or chicken pox. However, physical and emotional shocks also form tonic diseases. A contusion (bruise) is also always the same, as is a concussion. A shock related to a death of a loved one is equally constant in nature. Finally, we also have diseases caused by hemical toxins, including drugs. These diseases are hidden under the term "side-effects." This simply means that these are not the effects the chemical manufacturers want, but they are disease-effects nonetheless. The wonderful thing is that since the disease remains constant in nature, the medicine for the disease is also constant.

However, these tonic diseases can give rise to other diseases, which will depend on the time and circumstances of the case. These cannot be predicted or treated by knowing the cause (which is the tonic disease). You can only treat them by taking the symptoms produced and then matching this disease picture with the picture produced by a medicine. We call these pathic diseases (from the term "pathos" which means "suffering"). The good news is that by treating for the tonic diseases, many of the pathic diseases also are destroyed, but occasionally a pathic disease remains to be identified and removed.

Let's take a simple case of a child who is exposed to chicken pox and then comes down with the characteristic symptoms of this disease. Knowing it is chicken pox, we can give the child the specific medicine for chicken pox, which happens to be a highly diluted and potentized remedy made from the chicken pox virus (this *is* a disease-causing microbe, after all!). There is no longer any virus left in the solution, but only the energetic vibration of the virus. This is enough, because the life force of the patient acts as if it was being given the virus. According to the natural law of similar resonance, the medicine destroys the disease (two similar energetic patterns will destroy each other). The child may recover right away, or, in a more extreme case, there may be some symptoms that linger. We can analyze all these symptoms and then find a remedy that has the same symptom picture.

To find disease pictures or images, we give healthy volunteers a highly diluted and dynamized substance and then record what happens. We call these tests *provings*. Remember, each substance has a potential effect on our life force. Since the substance is really in an energetic form, it cannot create any lasting effects in the healthy person. You have probably carried out a similar proving, inadvertently, when you cut up an onion – watery eyes, itching and runny nose. These are symptoms similar to some allergic reactions, and potentized onion (*Allium cepa*) is a well-known remedy in homeopathy that works on allergy and hayfever symptoms that are similar to those produced when cutting up an onion.

The law of similars works everywhere in disease. You may have heard of its use in frostbite, where you are advised to use snow to gradually unfreeze the frozen part. To use heat (the law of opposites) would result in damage to the tissue.

It works equally in the case of burns, though we are taught, strangely enough, not to use it. Next time you have a burn, try the law of similars. When you use cold, you get instant relief, but as soon as you remove the cold, the burned part starts to hurt and you can often get scarring afterwards for a long time. When you use heat, you will notice an immediate increase in pain, followed very quickly by an ending of pain and the quick recovery of the skin. I recently spilled some scalding hot tea water over my arm in a restaurant. I didn't have any remedies with me, but remembered the law of similars and took my quite warm mug and placed it against my burned arm for as long as I could tolerate and did this several times.

Almost within a minute, the pain was gone and within about 30 minutes the angry red scar had disappeared.

The key, of course, is to remember the term "similar." If you use the same heat as caused the burn in the first place, you only get more of a burn. So, you have to use something less hot, but similar! It works. Years ago, I remember listening to a blacksmith explain how he treated burns (of which he received many), which was to put his burned part as close to the fire as he could stand. He stated that this way it healed quickly and left no scarring. His arms were indeed devoid of scars. People were impressed, but no one understood why, as this went against the "official" advice.

We are also told to use cold packs when we have inflammation (swelling), such as occurs when we get a serious sprain or strain, but the law of similars would demand heat. Strangely enough, this is what we do when we lightly strain our muscles, but when there is visible swelling, it seems conventional medicine doesn't trust the body's healing power and tries to suppress the evidence. Inflammation and heat is the way the body heals.

THE THREE REALMS OF MEDICINE

Any system of medicine has three realms or divisions:

1. Therapeutic Regimen (diet, nutrition, lifestyle) – restoration of balance when the state of health is temporarily disturbed

2. Therapeutic Medicine Proper – cure of disease

3. Therapeutic Education – providing meaning for one's journey through life

I'd like to give you an outline of each of these in Heilkunst.

Therapeutic Regimen

There is a lot of advice out there about what to do and what not to do to remain healthy. Who to believe? First, it is important to determine jurisdiction. In human law, the issue of jurisdiction is the first thing considered. If you live in one state or province, the laws of another state or province don't apply to you. If you have committed an offence under federal law, then only federal courts and judges have jurisdiction over the case.

When you are a practitioner, you are detective, arresting officer, prosecutor, judge and jury, and bailiff all rolled into one. You have to determine if you have jurisdiction over the case (does it fall within your area of competence?) before you can act. You also have to decide in which court the case is to be tried (treated). If it is a case of simple imbalance, not drinking enough water for example, or not getting enough exercise, then you can't take it to Medical Court; it has to be tried in Regimenal Court.

Regimen is the realm of imbalance or illness that is simply due to a lack or excess of something. It is easily corrected, because it has only disturbed the sustentive power of our living principle, the Dynamis. The natural law that applies here is the law of opposites. If you determine that a patient has not been getting enough of the right kind of nutrients, for example, or has an energy imbalance, then the sentence of the court (diagnosis) is clear. The patient must, to regain health, start eating the right nutrients or have the energy imbalance corrected. To not do so would be a contempt of court (in this case an offence against natural law). The only punishment meted out in the case of a failure to follow the sentence of the court is one that you inflict on yourself – continued ill-health.

How do you tell what are the right kind of nutrients for a person, or the best way to correct an energy imbalance? Heilkunst provides the principles that tell you what is right for your type or for your condition. For example, if you have had a difficult birth, then the use of one of several manipulative methods, such as osteopathy, cranio-sacral therapy or chiropractic to correct the distortion in the cranium and spine, is warranted. If you are a particular blood type, have a particular dominant endocrine gland and have a certain metabolic type (all of which are easily determined) then the particular foods, supplements and exercises that are right for you will be known.

Therapeutic Medicine Proper

If, however, you have acquired a disease, then the problem will not be fixed by any judgment from the Regimenal Court. Disease involves an impingement or damage to the generative power that can only be corrected by the application of the law of similars. No amount of right diet or energy work will remove the fact that you have a given disease. Regimen can make you feel better and stronger, but the disease will continue to grow.

Remember the woman I mentioned earlier who had found relief from her symptoms from regimenal measures? She found that the symptoms eventually came back and that she felt worse than before. Why? Because the disease increased and continue to weaken her constitution and eventually overcame her system despite all the good things she was doing for her health.

Disease needs to be prosecuted in front of a judge that has jurisdiction over the natural law of similars. Then, after the proper trial, the right sentence can be pronounced and the guilty properly dealt with. In this case it is not the fault of the patient as in regimen. The guilty party is the disease, which must be identified and then removed. If the headache is caused by a concussion from a fall, then it can only, and must, be removed by the application of a medicine chosen on the basis of the law of similars.

In this case, it must be a medicine that has the power to cause in a healthy person the same symptom, even though they have not had a concussion (but it's as if they had – the law of similars). Again, the judgment of the court can be ignored, but the result is simply more suffering.

Therapeutic Education

Much of our ill health and disease arises from ignorance. Since we cannot abide a pure state of ignorance, we have to fill in the vacuum of knowledge with a belief. If the belief is understood as a temporary (and not necessarily true) explanation of reality, we have an hypothesis and we have science. If a belief is treated as being true, even in the face of evidence to the contrary and any challenge of the belief is met with emotional reactions or attacks on the messenger, we have superstition and false belief.

False belief leads eventually to false thinking, which in turn leads to customs and traditions that are then the means to inculcate subsequent generations in the false belief. It is a self-perpetuating system.

The only remedy here is truth. This is a tricky issue, as we are all subject to error. However, this is not to say that we cannot know the truth. Truth comes from our deeper, inner knowing, from the realm of cosmic wisdom that we were given on birth. Truth is more a matter of recognition than of learning something new. A teacher is a guide to our own discovery of this inner wisdom and helps us to bring it into our consciousness so that it doesn't just remain as a feeling or "gut instinct."

Science is now talking about the discovery of a brain that is more complex and has more nerve endings than our brain mind. This other brain is situated in our solar plexus or gut. When we know something we feel a sense of recognition of self and connection to the universe that gives us peace of mind. We are not upset when this knowing is challenged, for our knowing is not a belief, uncertain and open to doubt. We do not have to have others agree with it, as truth is not a matter of how many people support it. Even if no one agrees with us, it remains the truth.

My mother taught me about this other brain and this other way of knowing. She has an unerring instinct about people and events; she could even tell what sex a person's baby would be. She is just matter of fact and calm about what she knows and isn't too concerned whether others agree or not. "I know what I know," she will say. My father is more the intellectual side of knowing, seeing everything rationally and being able to explain the logic of things. He knows a tremendous amount of history, geography, politics and language (in fact, that is where I got most of my formal education), but he isn't as worldly-wise as my mother.

We've all had "aha" moments, those Eureka experiences when we "got" something, or when a solution to a problem presented itself to us. This is the well-spring of all creativity. Science is built by geniuses, who are geniuses precisely because they can, more so than most of us, tap into this deep, inner knowing of all things and then present it to the world as a gift in the form of a new insight or a new machine or device to make life easier (and more complicated, too!). We all have this genial capacity, except that we either don't listen to it, or don't do anything specific with it.

Yet, we can develop our ability to tap into this capacity. Disease shuts us off from this ability, particularly chronic disease, which is why we tend to call it "degenerative," because it weakens our generative or creative power. So, health in terms of freedom from chronic disease is a precondition for the constructive and rational use of our inner genius. Most natural genius, if not in a healthy person, tends to be destructive (mad scientist) or self-destructive (mad artist). Like the energy of an exuberant and active teenager, it needs to be channelled into constructive pursuits.

So a large part of becoming healthy, and of any system that tries to bring a person to health, must be the ability to develop our organs of inner knowledge, and the ability to make sense of this new world. We have to live in this world of matter and the external senses, but we also need to integrate our inner knowing with our outer world – this is true science.

This is precisely what Heilkunst does – it brings us into contact with our inner self, through a journey into our past traumas, to retrieve and bring into the whole various parts of our soul that have been left stranded in time (for example, at age eight when we had a severe emotional shock). In a sense, you can travel back into time. While your physical body remains behind, your energetic and soul bodies can actually time travel.

Part of this past we have to overcome and transform comes from the events in this lifetime, but it is clear that part of it comes in with us when we are born. We definitely know that there is a genetic inheritance of conditions, even diseases such as syphilis or TB. This is on the natural or earth side of our being, the side of the Dynamis. There is also growing evidence that we have a different kind of inheritance, one that comes from the side of Spirit (Spiritus). This is the origin of many of our spiritual diseases, involving ignorance and false beliefs. Any true medical system has to address both the natural and the spiritual diseases, which is what Heilkunst does.

This brings us to a very difficult question, namely why do we get sick, or ultimately, "why do bad things happen to good people?" The answer partly is given in those accounts by remarkable people who tell of their struggle with a serious illness or disease and how it has altered their life for the better. It comes in the changed lives people lead after a near-death experience.

Illness and disease are adversaries that we have to test ourselves against. They all have meaning if we are open to receiving it. While no one would wish an illness or disease on anyone, we cannot deny that disease has the power to alter our lives. While we may say that we like or dislike something or that it is either pleasant or unpleasant, we cannot really say that something is "bad" or "good" in a moralistic way, for that is to judge, which is the province of a higher power than us. If I look back on my life, I have to admit that the experiences that were most challenging and unpleasant are also the ones that changed me the most, for the better. As my parents would say, adversity builds character. As humans we have a tendency to remain static, to desire only the one side of things, usually the sweet side. We don't like the bitter, but as any herbalist will tell you, too much sweet disturbs the digestion – a little bit of bitter will set things right again.

The world is built around polarities. We have both a spirit and a dynamic pole within us. We have both a generative and a sustentive power within our Dynamis. We cannot know light unless we also know dark. Of course, light will always overcome dark, but to become light it has to have the dark. Indeed, as the German scientist, Goethe, showed us and as any artist knows (and contrary to what Newton taught), colour emerges out of the interplay of light and dark. In fact, the sky is blue because that is the colour produced when pure light (sunlight) is seen against a pure dark background (space). Also, the colours in the morning sky (blue spectrum) are produced when the light meets the dark and the colours of the sunset are produced when the dark comes to meet the light (red spectrum).

We cannot know health without knowing illness or disease. Illness and disease are like confinements or prisons. They restrict our freedom as human beings. We cannot really be free if we have not first known imprisonment. And we cannot be truly free unless that struggle is one that we overcome. Others can help us, but we need to do it for ourselves. The fight against illness and disease is a very personal struggle, one that is very lonely, but one that has the ability also to set us free spiritually.

Thus, it is hard to say that disease is "bad" in a moral sense. It is simply an adversary, which is the meaning of the term Satan in scripture. We can and must struggle against illness and disease. That is our responsibility, for it is also the path to freedom as human beings. Freedom means having a sense of inner joy and calm that comes from knowing ourselves, and from knowing that the world and its experiences are not punishments or rewards from capricious gods, but simply a gigantic stage for finding ourselves. We learn to be free of fear and learn to love ourselves and the world with all its imperfections, and to trust that what is, is what must be for our spiritual journey - but also what can be changed by our own creative power.

In its deepest sense, we discover that the world is but a reflection of our state of mind and that if we change this, the world changes. I remember a patient who complained that no one loved her, that everyone was always abandoning her. She eventually discovered that she had a belief that no one could love her because she was not worthy of any love. When she became healthy enough to acknowledge this belief and overcome the fear of challenging it, she discovered that the world is indeed full of love. She found a resonant intimate relationship with someone who reflected her unconditional love and acceptance of herself. Previous lovers could never love her enough, because she could never trust their love so long as she believed that she was not worthy of being loved. Eventually, they left her and she was confirmed in her belief, a self-fulfilling prophecy. This only deepened her sense of failure and unworthiness. Now, instead, she has a sense of trust in love and a sense that the world is built on love. She can see in the difficult passages the love of the universe pressing us to explore our inner selves and to come into our own power and light.

It is hard to tell someone who is suffering that this is a necessary part of life and that it actually has universal love behind it. However, from a spiritual perspective, this is indeed the case. We achieve freedom when we understand that the energy that drives the universe of the Creator is love and that all that is, is neither good nor bad, but are experiences designed to help us unfold who we are. Thus, it is not that bad things happen to good people, but that *things* happen to people and we have to trust that there is a deeper spiritual purpose behind *all* events even if we cannot see what that might be, particularly through our pain.

Medicine is a gift from the Creator that allows us to remove suffering much faster than might otherwise be the case, but also to tackle deep issues that we might not have been strong enough to handle. Spiritual growth is like human.

As we mature, we are given more and more responsibility along with our freedom. In our work we also undertake greater responsibility and challenges as we grow in our experience and abilities.

However, medicine must act according to natural law, otherwise it will lead to harm, no matter how much good it appears to be doing. Of course, there is a place for surgery, antibiotics and chemical drugs, but they must be used within their jurisdiction. Heilkunst includes a role for these but it is limited and severely restricted. To use them routinely and repeatedly in other than severe emergencies where the life force is almost gone, is to harm.

To use medicine outside of natural law principles and jurisdiction is also to suppress the spiritual path that each person has before them. We must go to meet our suffering and then, with the aid of medicine acting lawfully, to transform it, not hide from it or suppress it. If we follow natural and spiritual law, as is the case in Heilkunst, we achieve spiritual growth and true inner peace and knowing. We come to live fully in the world, yet to act according to the dictates of our deep, inner knowing and desire or love. We live in unconditional love and follow that love where it resonates so that we experience deep fulfillment, a treasure and wealth that is beyond measure and that cannot be taken away by anyone.

Chapter Two

A Long Road Home
A Physician's Journey from West to East and Back Again

By Leonard Levine, MD, DPH, CCFP, DAc, FCFP(C), FRCP(MA)

About Leonard Levine

Born and raised in St. John, New Brunswick, Dr. Levine completed medical school at Dalhousie University in Halifax and postgraduate studies in Toronto. His healing knowledge expanded considerably when he spent time with various healers and teachers in various places abroad such as India and Tibet.

In his medical practice today, Dr. Levine incorporates a wide range of therapies including homeopathy, acupuncture, diet, vitamin/mineral supplements and assorted stress reduction techniques. He firmly believes in people's power to heal themselves and the medical doctor's role as assistant in that process.

Dr. Levine has worked diligently to expand the traditional western medical paradigm. He was president of the Canadian Wholistic Medical Association and is considered an expert in the field.

Currently enhancing his knowledge further by studying at the Hahnemann Center for Heilkunst, Dr. Levine lives in the quiet town of Pakenham, Ontario and enjoys life in semi-retirement.

A LONG ROAD HOME
A PHYSICIAN'S JOURNEY FROM WEST TO EAST AND BACK AGAIN

What a day this has been! I have just let a patient go from my practice. I am loath to do this, as this patient and her family have been involved in my practice for about 25 years. However, it seems that our ethos and direction have moved away from our original contract. The bigger the front, the bigger the back is an old macrobiotic expression. This lady originally came to my practice because of a sore back. We dealt with her and her family for many years. However, this morning our dialogue seemed to shift. Our original contract seemed to have been broken.

Hence, we parted company today and I feel a deep sense of loss because I become involved with my patients on many levels of body, mind and spirit. She seems to have gone the way of the drug route versus a natural herb, vitamin and homeopathic route. I am not against drugs – I don't throw the baby out with the bath water, but when someone makes excessive demands and wants to ride herd over me, something within rebels.

I am a compassionate physician and one who has a great deal of patience and willingness to look at alternative medicine and alternative therapies. In this day and this age of paradigm shifts, I have been experiencing a new thread in the practice of medicine.

One could ask how you will be different after reading this chapter? My reward or cue is spiritual. If anyone of you gets a flavour of how alternative/complementary medicine augments traditional western medicine, I will be ecstatic with joy.

Thus I shall present various scenarios and you can choose the outcome and your own direction or path. This chapter is meant to stir you on a course for your own growth. It will enhance your inner voice speaking through you.

THE EARLY YEARS

My interest in medicine began many years ago. As a child in St. John, New Brunswick; New Waterford, Nova Scotia; Orlando, Florida; and lastly in Moncton, New Brunswick, I gleaned a wealth of experience from a varied background. My grandmother had an incredible effect on me, as did my internship in St. John's, Newfoundland.

My grandmother, a Russian-Ukrainian lady grew up in Rovnia in the Belarus Country. As a child, her way to health was complemented with the use of many natural substances, which were found in a small Russian schtettle (village). In fact, often when a doctor could not be found, a fever treated with Yarrow, Willow Bark, Mustard Poultice or Liniment solved the problem and at the same time, saved lives.

My grandmother used all of these old fashioned remedies and I include my remedy sheet for your perusal (see Table 1). It was first published many years ago in the *Journal of the College of Family Physicians of Canada*. Take a look and you will see many of your own folk remedies there. For example, I am sure that you grew up knowing that gargling with salt water or honey tea and lemon were valuable remedies for the common cold.

These early years were formative for me. I became instilled with an attitude as well as a spirit of self-sufficiency. In the 1940s and 50s, no one ran to the doctor. We asked our grandparents and family members what to do and usually an old fashioned remedy was suggested.

Boy Scouts, baseball, picking blueberries, selling Christmas trees and Christmas candies kept me busy in my early years. My dad had a grocery store in Moncton and I used to work in the vegetable room as well as the meat room. In fact, I remember my dad's first grocery store in St. John, New Brunswick. In 1943, the floor in the

Table 1: GRANDMOTHER'S REMEDY SHEET

Colds
Vitamin C
Orange juice
Tea and Lemon
Honey and Lemon
Gargle Salt Water
Sniff Salt Water
Goose Grease
Camphorated Oil

Stomach Cramps
Cinnamon Tea
Ginger Tea

Diarrhea
Buttermilk
Yogurt

Diarrhea and Vomiting
Combine:
8 oz flat Cola
4 tsp Sugar
1 tsp Salt
1 tsp Baking Soda
Add water to make one quart

Nausea
Rice Water Soup
Grated Apple
(Browned)

Kidneys
Bread and Milk
Cranberry Juice
Corn Silk

Accidents
Massage, Ice
Physiotherapy
Exercise, Yoga
Epsom Salt Compress
K-Fong Yeow

Nerves
Salads
Sunflower Seeds

Constipation
Prunes, Dates, Figs
Pumpkin Seeds

Temperatures
Sponge Bath (tepid water)
Alcohol Sponge
Bath (water and alcohol)
Fan over Sheet

Insomnia
Hot Bath
Hops Tea
Celestial Tea
Massage

Skin Rashes
Oatmeal Bath

Ingredients for Poultices
Pollen
Linseed Meal
Onion and Garlic
Mustard Plaster
Parsnip Water

meat cutting room was covered with sawdust. The sawdust was collected and disposed of each day. Later on in his grocery store in Moncton, New Brunswick, this "unsanitary" practice was scorned as unwholesome by the health authorities. By today's standards it probably was.

I remember one of Dad's employees sliced his hand and Dad immediately applied an ice-cold steak bound with a white rag as a compression bandage to quell the bleeding. They rushed him to the Moncton Hospital. That was in 1952. I can still see the blood flowing and oozing through the bandage, yet he came out just fine. Antibiotics were coming into vogue, but Doctor Allan Hopper did not use any at this time because there was no infection to treat.

During my high school years, I had a yearning to be involved in medicine. I guess it all began in 1951 when I was out hunting. I shot a robin with a beebee gun. This was not a good practice, but kids will be kids. That was a traumatic experience for me, not to mention the robin. I watched the robin slowly die. When he finally closed his eyes, I vowed to spend my life helping and healing people.

First aid courses and school years kept me busy and my family doctor, Dr. Allan Hopper, of Moncton put the "bee in my bonnet" to study medicine. I enjoyed my first aid studies taught by Charlie Paul of the Moncton corps of the St. John Ambulance. Dr. Allan Hopper was my teacher. He also taught me stargazing, and always said to reach for the skies.

Thus my aspiration to become a physician was born. High school led me on to pre-med, medical school and medical practice. At times I was scared to death, but gradually I began to feel confident. Dalhousie University in Halifax, Nova Scotia gave us excellent preparation. Graduating in 1967, I went west as a lot of young men do, and moved to Toronto. My early years in practice and post-graduate training at Women's College Hospital created in me a yen to travel. I felt that I had learned so much in Medical School and I wanted to share some of these gifts with other people.

DISCOVERING ANCIENT HEALING

My travels began. After practice in Toronto with Dr. Norm Angel, and a locum study period at Toronto's psychiatric hospital at 999 Queen Street, I scooted off to India in July 1971 to work with the Tibetan refugees. A cholera epidemic in

Bangladesh was my reason to explore. For political reasons, Bangladesh did not materialize but I was given an opportunity to travel with a Tibetan witch doctor, the Nagpa from Ragpur. We went from patient to patient "exorcising demons." I traveled through India with a group of people from many different countries. It was exciting and spiritually awakening.

In India I was exposed to many ancient arts of Tibetan medicine – Ayurvedic medicine, herbs, gems, stones and magic. I saw men being hung up with needles through their skin, people walking on hot coals, and Tibetan lamas performing celebrations in Dharmasala, Calcutta, Darjeeling and Sikkim. The rickshaws of Calcutta and Delhi were often my way of transportation. Setting up clinics to see patients in little hubbles or in the backs of monasteries or high in the Himalayas was my manner of practice.

From India to Canada I flew. I worked another year to earn money and return once again in 1972/73. I wished to work in the Himalayas. India, Africa, South East Asia, Australia and New Zealand provided my teachers. The Aboriginals in Australia, the healing Dukuns of Bali and the Fakirs of Indonesia all taught me a "new," yet truly very old, medicine.

Homeopathy, an established art in India, yielded some remarkable cures for the natives of Delhi and Bombay. I watched skilled Indian homeopaths work their miracles with little white pellets. Truly, I thought it was some kind of hocus-pocus at first and then I began to see marvellous results.

My return to Canada heralded another paradigm shift. I could feel myself changing and witnessed phenomenal results in the 70s when I began to practise acupuncture.

Surgery, psychotherapy and prescription medications such as antibiotics provide the traditional physician with the tools of his trade, thus when I first watched and studied acupuncture in Bali, Indonesia in 1972, I was given a nudge into a new direction for my practice of medicine. Meridians, energy and energy-chi became another language for me to familiarize and become comfortable with. Shen-men (spirit door) opened a new vista for me as I began my initial departure from the western paradigm. Acupuncture in the early '70s was looked upon as a placebo until the scientific discovery of endorphins was postulated and proven by Dr. Bruce

Pomerantz, a physician and researcher with the department of zoology at the University of Toronto.

Please join me as I share with you some of the fascinating healing that I observed once I started to incorporate some of these teachings in my work.

While I was practising in Crete in 1975, a patient, Scott H., came to see me at our clinic in Paleohora. He had a huge abscess on his left elbow. I had no antibiotics or local anaesthetic with me. By inserting six acupuncture needles into very important points, I was able to anesthetise Scott's arm and lance his abscess with very little pain. I incised and drained the abscess and he was most grateful.

Returning home to Canada in mid 1973, I was called to see Penny C., a 12-year-old pre-teen at the emergency department at the Strathroy Middlesex Hospital near London, Ontario. The emergency room was full with overflow patients lined up on all the stretchers. Her dad gave me permission to do acupuncture to stop her pain. She had a green stick fracture of the left forearm. Inserting eight needles and waiting 20 minutes allowed me to manipulate, set the fracture and put it in a plaster of Paris cast. She experienced no pain. I sent her home to Arkona, Ontario with some prescription pain medication. Not only was I able to set the fracture with the acupuncture, but it also seemed as if she healed more rapidly than might otherwise have been expected.

I asked her dad to apply a ceramic bar magnet over the cast fracture site to facilitate healing and diminish the pain. It worked. In addition, her dad, an electrician, had heard that an extension cord, wrapped around the fracture site six to seven times, with one end plugged into the wall socket and the other end plugged into a lamp would also speed the healing. She kept company with a 40-watt light bulb for 20 minutes a day while the magnet, electricity plus continued acupuncture helped heal the break.

Certainly magnetism, acupuncture and electrical healing are departures from traditional therapy, yet over the years, I have found these alternative therapies quite effective.

Dorothy G., an arthritic lady in her 70s, began to smile and was pain-free only a few minutes after I inserted just four needles into her body. Was this magical, was it placebo, or was it real? You be the judge. I know what I think.

In 1977, further education resulting in a Public Health Diploma eased me into another shift in medicine. I came to believe that the use of preventive medicine on a clinical level would begin to eliminate people's poor habits and help them change.

PHYSICIAN HEAL THYSELF

What a surprise I was in for! Before I could incorporate any more new techniques into my practice, I had to change my habits first. As the universe would have it, I got ill with a brain tumour and was given six months to live. I was devastated and shocked.

Thankfully, I remembered the Nagpa's advice, "Go the hills and clear thy soul." I did! Off to a monastery in Kinmount, Ontario I went. I meditated, walked in the forest, ate wholesome food and rested. I'm not sure to this day just what happened, but gradually I regained my energy and the retreat to nature seemed to return me to health. I was ready to re-enter medical practice, and moved to Ottawa, Ontario. That was almost 30 years ago, and there has been no sign of the tumour since.

YOU ARE WHAT YOU EAT

In Ottawa my practice of wholistic medicine began with a plunge into the nutritional aspect of medical practice. Yes vitamins, herbs and minerals along with clinical scientific laboratory testing became another avenue to entice, spur and motivate my patients.

Irena J., a 30-year-old Polish woman presented to my office with severe facial acne. Each visit, she came armed with pencil and paper and made voluminous notes. She got onto a yeast-free diet, cutting out the ABC's (alcohol, bread, candy, coffee, colas and cookies), and added vitamins including high potency vitamin A therapy. Over the next seven months, she modified her diet and was rewarded with clear, unblemished skin and remarkably improved health. To this day I still see her and her family for their regular health maintenance.

Mary T., a 38-year-old petite brunette, had been having joint pains in her fingers and wrists. Her mom had had the same symptoms at the same time in her life. After checking Mary for allergies, I removed dairy and wheat products from her diet and substituted goat's milk and rye crackers. Vitamins, particularly calcium, magnesium, vitamin C and zinc were added to her diet and she seemed to make significant improvement within a month and a half. She returned for some acupuncture and continued with the hypoallergenic diet and did quite well. She told her mom about the therapy and they both are much better now.

Stephan L., a 42-year-old civil servant from Quebec came to my office with attention deficit disorder. He was speaking so fast, and was filled with such uncontrollable anxiety that he could not sit still and kept running around from chair to chair, room to room, just trying to get comfortable. I did some acupuncture on him to calm him down before our consultation. Acupuncture, meditation, vitamins and psychotherapy brought much peace to his life, and to this day, he still has benefits from his acupuncture and proper nutrition.

Morley M., 42, was a severely ill schizophrenic who came to my office in February 1981. He was exhibiting very dysfunctional behaviour; hearing voices, seeing visions and arguing with his 78-year-old mother. I did not cure his schizophrenia, but with acupuncture, talk therapy, medication and vitamins, he improved remarkably. His good friend Bill M. and I still have a great chuckle when we talk about him. Unfortunately, our good friend passed away and will not get a chance to see his name in print. He was a magnanimous, funny person, a real character. I will miss him.

The old expression of walk tall and carry a big stick is one that I began to follow. The big stick was not a cudgel but merely an empowerment for my patients to see health as a commodity of wellness. I give them full credit, for they taught me the value of good food, good air, good water, exercise and persistence. I saw miracles happen in front of me as people who had been ill for years somehow made marvellous recoveries.

In 1980, I joined the practice of Dr. L. Gilka and was motivated to further my studies of alternative medicine. She instructed and supported me in my undertaking in the study of nutrition, allergies and the use of enzyme-enhancing agents. As well, we looked at the function of convenience foods as causation for illness. Dr. Gilka, a well-known alternative Ottawa physician, deserves much credit for the spread of alternative medicine in the Ottawa Valley, for she has helped many patients in putting them on the right path. We continue to be great friends and colleagues to this day.

Henrietta R., an 82-year-young Dutch lady came to see me in 1984 with extremely swollen legs and severe arthritis. She was experiencing heart failure and to boot, was hard of hearing. Believe me, it was difficult taking a history and doing an examination. She was a very knowledgeable woman and would come to my office with many old-fashioned remedies, which she carried with her from Indonesia and Holland. Poultices of cabbage leaves, aloe vera and alfalfa were often deposited at my feet as she pleaded with me, "Please, Dr. Levine, use these on your patients." She came with paper bags and shopping bags and different potions in small, non-descript vials and asked me to solve the mystery of her health conundrums. We dialogued monthly for several years, and finally, as she solved her health problems and educated me in the finer healing arts of the far east, she carried on remarkably well, well into her 90s. What an interesting human being she was!

HOMEOPATHY AND HEILKUNST

Through the '80s and '90s we wholistic doctors were able to make significant impact on our patient base and they on us. This enabled another shift to happen and during a Naturopathic Program, which I undertook at the Ontario College of Naturopathic Medicine (OCNM), Drs. Greg Hershoff and John Laplante began to point out the value of those little pellets, those little white pills that I had seen in India. Homeopathy was reborn in me once again. I knew that this was a method which had to be resurrected in the west as a bona fide healing modality.

I learned that these little white pellets had a phenomenal impact on people. I watched skilled Canadian practitioners use these homeopathic medicines, but I was not convinced. I did not yet have either the skill or the intense concentration and perseverance to do homeopathic medicine. But time held me in her arms and I began to see the power of these little pills. Over the years I have come to understand what I did not comprehend in my early years of study, even though I had studied with respected teachers such as Drs. Buko, Levy, Jayasuriya and Des Payne. Diligence, persistence and knowledge come with the tincture of time and respect.

Somehow in my medical training I had been so indoctrinated that I could not see beyond Avogadro's number ($6x10^{23}$). Avogadro's number is a quantifying number beyond which no original molecules of a substance can be detected or measured. I could not understand how these minute amounts of a substance, added to distilled water and potentized by shaking and secussion (smacking the bottle vigorously about a dozen times against the palm of the hand), could actually cure illness. I slowly began to comprehend that there really was no scientific explanation for homeopathy yet, but I began to look at it another way, to view it from a different angle. I had to take a quantum leap in consciousness that in a sense was a huge leap of faith.

An article by Benveniste, a French scientist, appeared in *Nature Magazine.* His understanding of the action of homeopathic medicine was based on physics and quantum mechanics, so I propelled my consciousness into another level of awareness. Still I was puzzled. I could not wrap my mind around or even introduce my mind to a concept of supersensible causation.

I began to study Heilkunst with Rudi Verspoor, and another paradigm shift happened. I felt as if I was in a different dimension as Rudi introduced the ideas of Heilkunst to me. Hahnemann's *Organon* interpreted by Decker and Verspoor threw open the doors of my mind. These teachers shined light in the crevasses, which heretofore had been in the penumbra of darkness.

JACQUELINE

Usually people come to me through referrals from other patients, friends or clinicians, or I just might meet somebody over lunch and get into a dialogue. Life is everywhere and so is illness and health. I do not make any exceptions or distinctions. Life is about love and one needs to love oneself as well as one's patients.

Like heals like is one of the rules of homeopathy. I do not mean that you have to be in love with your patients, I mean that the state of love is manifest. One is not clinging to loving someone or holding on to someone, one merely exudes that flavour of loving-kindness. As a practising Jewish Buddhist, I know that the torah inculcates the lessons of Buddhism. Strange as it may seem, both teach right action, right livelihood and wholesome and nourishing thoughts.

While leaving Rudi Verspoor's office one day, I bumped into an old acquaintance, Jacqueline. Having not seen each other for seven years, we decided to go for a cup of tea. We chose to meet at a lovely restaurant in Manotick, Oggi's. What a beautiful setting! It was early September, five or five thirty in the afternoon and we enjoyed one of the last meals to be served outside that day. From this beautiful evening and reintroduction to each other, we decided to meet again and discuss the facets of doing a project together. But one very interesting thing happened during our meeting. Jacqueline's cell phone rang. It was her husband. He was wondering where she was and whether she was coming home for dinner. The moment Jacqueline picked up the phone, I noticed that her facial tone and colour suddenly became piqued, and her voice went down a total octave in timbre. She became depressed. I felt her energy shift as she became meek and depleted right before my eyes. I could sense her ambivalence and her reticence to talk with her husband.

After she hung up, I told Jacqueline that whoever was on the other line was sucking her energy and not feeding her. I knew that she needed to disconnect from this other person. Was I reading too much into a conversation? Was I making too much from a change in the quality and timbre of a dialogue?

What I experience in participating people is that I must trust my inner voice and intuition. My intuition here told me that Jacqueline was in an unwholesome, ungiving, unnourishing relationship, and if she were to continue, her health would deteriorate. That I was sure of! The next time I met Jacqueline, she had a cracked rib on the left side, and the meeting after that, she burned her hand. What an incredible litany of symptoms and occurrences! Was it synchronicity, or was the universe just talking to Jacqueline through me?

In any case, her level of well-being had been interfered with and was still in process of acting out. True to my professional standards, I never mentioned to Jacqueline my thoughts about her marriage. I did not encourage her one way or the other. I never mentioned her relationship again after that first observation at Oggi's. However, after she cracked her rib and burned her hand, I began to address issues that were and had been on my mind. With her permission, I asked if she would like to review the many facets of her life — body, mind and spirit. Thankfully for Jacqueline, by this time, she had already left the one-year marriage that had been draining her so much.

While Jacqueline's new home was being readied, Jacqueline moved in with her daughter for two weeks. This brought out other unexpected opportunities for healing.

It was during our second meeting at another restaurant, the Rooster Roadhouse in Carp, Ontario, that Jacqueline happened to mention that she had fallen down and hurt her ribs on the left chest. As usual, when somebody tells me a complaint of any sort, my computer-like mind begins to look at the many parameters of that complaint. Thus, I began to ask Jacqueline about herself. This was a bruise under her left breast and ribs, which occurred when she jammed her left elbow into the left chest. She had fallen while talking on her cell phone. Holding the cell phone in her left hand, she had tripped on the curb of the sidewalk, and had fallen, jabbing her elbow into her ribs. As a medical doctor, I look at the anatomical shifts happening and the emotional components, yet from a Heilkunst point of view, my mind veers off in a different direction. Left side of the body, menopausal years, relationships, and my mind jumps into a total new parameter of understanding. I began to ask Jacqueline some very personal questions, which at first went beyond the simple anatomical problem to the emotional and psychological facets of her personality.

In Heilkunst, as in western medicine, asking questions is a must. We always look beyond the more subtle to get to the more complex, and Jacqueline obviously had some complex problems to deal with. While sitting with her at the Rooster Roadhouse, I also noticed that her facial skin was dry. She had some wrinkles on her face and some crow's-feet at the side of her eyes.

I asked her if I could press at the junction of the breastbone and ribs. This is called the costal-chondral junction. I pressed and she winced. This is a clinical sign. It indicates a syndrome called Tietz Syndrome. Tietz syndrome may happen in menopausal women and may indicate an imbalance in calcium/magnesium, and may also indicate inflammation at other joints in her body. I informed Jacqueline that we were looking at the musculo-skeletal system as well as the integumentary system (skin, muscles and bones). I would need to do a physical examination to ascertain which vitamins she required, which minerals and herbs she needed, and what other nutrients she would need from her food.

Usually in my first visit with a client or patient, I do a history of the present illness, a history of past health (family history) and a functional inquiry to determine what is wrong. So I asked Jacqueline a series of questions and got a list of about 30 symptoms, surprising for a woman who is a healthy vegetarian, exercises at least five times a week, never gets colds, and considers herself in good health. Something was showing itself to me that needed healing and I informed Jacqueline that if she would like, we could do some lab tests, look at a nutritional history, do a physical examination, and follow up this visit with further investigation. The investigation was to be not only of herself, but also of her relationships with her family of origin, with her husband and with her children.

THE BURN

Two weeks later, Jacqueline came again to interview me about my practice. We had just started when she inadvertently poured scalding water over her right hand, her working hand.

We immediately stopped our discussion and began to put action to the words; walk the talk, so to speak. The regular western way of treating a first-degree burn, which is what she had, is to immerse the hand in cold water in an attempt to reduce the pain. As well, aspirin or other analgesics such as Anacin or Bufferin could be given to ameliorate the pain.

Jackie asked me to interpret this episode from my usual treatment method using western medicine versus how I would handle it from the point of view of Heilkunst. As I said, the western way would be to put the hand under ice-cold water for 3-5 minutes, add aspirin and then put on some Telfa and antibiotic ointments. I would bind up the hand with a roll of Kling gauze, and put the arm in a sling. Of course there are other components of this; for example, making sure the tetanus is up to date and ensuring that the burn has not gone deeper into the second layer of the dermis.

Then I would usually bring the person back 2-3 days later and if there appeared to be any blistered or elevated skin, I might remove the loose skin with a sterile procedure and once again apply a gauze soaked with antibiotic ointment such as Sofratulle and put on 4" by 4" gauze flats held in place with Kling.

I would follow this up for the next few days, attending to the scalded and burned area on the skin. If there were any suspicion of infection, I would take a swab, send it to the lab for analysis and follow this up if need be with an antibiotic, lotion, ointment or pills. The upshot of this process would be 3-4 weeks down the road, a possible scar on the back of Jacqueline's hand and another 4-5 weeks of healing.

So, what is the difference? How does Heilkunst treat Jacqueline's burn situation differently?

I immediately implemented one of the classical rules of homeopathy/ Heilkunst — *like treats like.* Jacqueline burned her hand. Since a burn is obviously heat, what do we do? We use heat to treat heat. I immediately took Jacqueline to the ladies' room and immersed her hand in hot water, which she said hurt like the dickens. Let us be sensible here, when I say hot water, to my hand, it did not feel hot, but since Jacqueline had burned her hand, the tissue had a memory of pain and was still in pain. So I started with lukewarm water to my touch, which she said felt hot and painful.

I held her hand in my hand and immersed both our hands in the lukewarm water and kept them there for 3-5 minutes. Then I continued to add hotter water from the tap, challenging both her and my sensitivities. I gradually increased the temperature of the water, until she felt the water was hot. As Jacqueline acclimatized to the hot water, I increased the temperature, yet her level of pain remained the same. After about 30 minutes of soaking both our hands in the hot water of increasing temperatures, we noticed that the colour of her hand, which had originally been very red, now diminished toward the natural colour of her other hand and became paler. Interestingly enough, her hand also felt cold to the touch at this time.

So slowly, as we soaked her hand in tepid then hotter water, there seemed to be a levelling of equilibrium between the temperature of the added hot water and the temperature of the burned hand. At the end of a half hour, the temperature felt much cooler, the redness had gone out of the skin, and there seemed to be some reduction in pain.

Simultaneously, at the moment of the burn, I had given Jacqueline the homeopathic remedy *Arnica* 30C. That was all I had in my bag. I then took Jacqueline with me to the Hahnemann Heilkunst Clinic on St. Joseph Blvd.

On the way over in the car, I phoned ahead to Venetia asking her to make up some drops of *Arnica* 10M, *Hypericum* 200M and *Cantharis* 1M. There are certain principles in the selection of these remedies, and these can be discussed at a later date. In my mind, the most important thing was to get the remedies to Jacqueline quickly, that is, in the first hour or so of her burning her hand. When we arrived at the clinic, Venetia had the remedies all ready for us, and Jacqueline immediately took 2-3 drops of the mixture. In addition, we used some *Calendula* ointment, which was applied to the back of her hand. No dressing was used. Jacqueline was advised to continue applying the ointment as needed, a very thin layer, over the next 2-3 hours and to continue taking the drops every 10-15 minutes.

This was continued over the next couple of days. On the first night, while lying in bed, Jacqueline could feel the covers touching the back of her hand. This caused a little discomfort, but not a lot. In fact, she was more concerned about the ointment rubbing off and staining the sheets than she was about the pain. By the second evening, she no longer felt the covers touching her hand and except for the feel of the ointment, she would have forgotten that she had a burn. There was no blistering, no redness and no heat. It was as if the skin on the back of the hand had forgotten that it had even been burned. "How magnificent, how amazing!" she said.

So you see, I have compared both methods, allopathic and homeopathic, and you can believe, that in my 30 years of practice, I have treated many burns equally and more serious than Jacqueline's. I have even worked in burn units in hospitals. This homeopathic treatment was wonderful!

A week later in my office, Jacqueline interviewed me and typed notes liberally on her laptop, without any sign of an injury. We are both thrilled that we can share with you this incident for it not only supports the view of the usefulness of Heilkunst in acute care, but also points the finger at the direction we could take with acute care medicine in the allopathic school. I daresay that in the treatment of burns and in burn units we most probably could reduce expenses by 7 to 10 percent and improve the quality and speed of healing by 85 to 90 percent. This could be accomplished by introducing the homeopathic remedies *Arnica, Hypericum* and *Cantharis* into burn units and using them liberally. There are homeopathic hospitals using these remedies in England, so why not here in Canada?

As she had been typing, I had been noticing that Jacqueline was wearing a tight purple turtleneck sweater. Not only was the turtleneck tight around her neck, but she also kept lifting it over her mouth and nose, covering three-quarters of her face. You must know that this is not an easy thing to do while you are typing, which shows how unconscious the movement was. I never just sit anywhere; I am always watching and diagnosing people, looking for clues to people's background and illnesses.

I told Jacqueline that her actions betrayed some facets of a remedy called *Lachesis*. I then read to her from the book *Leaders in Homeopathic Therapeutics* by E.B. Nash. Many of her symptoms can be found on pages 111 through 123. When I read to her from these pages, she suddenly had an epiphany. So much of her life, marriage, relationships and physical health were reflected on those pages.

Jacqueline went to her regular homeopathic practitioner to take the *Lachesis* and continue healing her life.

IN SUMMARY

Now, what do you think? Is there room for both of the above paths in medicine? Is there room for you to do the traditional orthodox medical treatment and at the same time incorporate the alternative practice?

Personally I have found that alternative/complementary medicine opens a totally new window of opportunity. It is as if I was given a second vision and totally new point of view.

Metaphorically speaking, if I were to imagine myself wearing a hockey helmet with a clear visor in front of it, much like Daniel Alfredsson wears when playing hockey for the Ottawa Senators, I would consider trying various different colours of visors to see how they improved or altered my vision.

Suppose I were wearing a dark visor and suddenly it was lifted and I was exposed to bright sunlight. For the first few moments I would feel dazed, and as my eyes and my brain adapted, there would gradually be some clearing. The brightness would gently disappear as my pupils accommodated.

This exciting process will happen to you as you open your mind to the possibilities of alternative medicine. Once you explore and put to the test various complementary/alternative methods, you will be divinely inspired to use other therapies. Exploring Heilkunst is much like pulling down a new visor with different colours, inculcating western modalities of healing while extending and complementing a new approach to the emotional modalities of wellness. Actually it is not new; for Hahnemann, the Father of Homeopathic Medicine, invented this discipline of therapy over 200 years ago.

It is only in the last 30 to 40 years that his methods are now being re-explored and taken out of the proverbial darkness. Remove the visor, expose the methods and modalities to modern scrutiny and we begin to open our minds to Hahnemann's discoveries.

I personally have been propelled by the results that my own patients have experienced. There is a Buddhist expression, "Ahe—posico," which means "put it to the test." Once you put your new experiences to the test with therapies, anything is possible.

Before I traveled the road to alternative medicine, I was a classical trained MD who got classical results in my practice of medicine. Statistically I would say this translated into a 35 to 40 percent success rate. After forging along in this new, complementary direction, I noticed a change. With my patients' help I was able to increase our success rate to 50 to 60 percent.

This is not bad considering that all I did was coach my patients with different views on nutrition, acupuncture, orthopedic medicine and Heilkunst. They have done "the work" and I have learned from our mutual experiences. This is not a singular approach, but a team approach, a team effort. We did the process and now we shall explore the outcome.

There is a high tech expression: "GI-GO" *Garbage in Garbage out.* Let's compare this with LI- LO. *Love in Love out.* Your visor can be your guide. The visor is analogous with your attitudes. As the Buddhists say, be positive and wholesome while you travel the right fold, noble path, and you will improve and get better.

Many people who came and consulted with me were in very poor physical health. The traditional medical treatment had failed them and they had been dejected by that failure. Standard medical practice had failed to heal. They were the rejects, the non- conformists, the rebels, but they had an open and inquiring mind and wished to be a part of the healing process. They did not want to be alienated from the process as happens in many of the western therapies.

We worked together and we all did our tasks; I did mine and they did theirs. Those who did not wish to comply nor work with me simply did not come back or continue the therapy of self-healing. Our path is the path less chosen. Many are called and few are chosen.

Introducing wholistic medicine into their lives opened them to a new and challenging adventure. Their role changed from that of a "dutiful child" to an active and scrutinizing participant. I watched many of them in my practice. I too have changed. I now see only eight to ten people per day as compared with 35 people per day. In my early career I used solutions which often proved to be temporary. Now I find using life-involving solutions much more satisfying.

Metaphorically speaking again, I moved from feeding them a fish to teaching them how to fish and find this much more challenging and adventuresome. After reading this book, I trust that you too will enjoy this new exploration and improve not only your health, but also your attitudes towards health.

Please remember, just reading is no panacea, for the road to Rome is paved with good intentions. Suffering (dukha) is part of the path to non-suffering. So please, be ye not deluded into the belief that after reading this chapter you have "the answer" to your health concerns. If just one of you... yes, maybe you... can experience a brief moment of epiphany in your own healing process, I will be thrilled and thank you for taking the time to assess and learn from this chapter.

Acknowledgements

April is the cruellest month
Lilacs out of the dead land, mixing
Memory and desire, stirring
Dull roots with spring rain.

– T.S. Elliot
The Waste Land

Serena Williamson is that essence of compassion and wholesome energy, which woke me from my lethargy and winter slumber and enabled me to put this chapter together. She lifted my spirit and nourished my psyche. She was the catalyst, the nucleus, the font of ideas and energy, which spearheaded this book, *Open Minds*, from our inner beings.

I am filled with gratitude and appreciation for her stimulus and support. If not for Serena, I would not have been able to complete this project. I am very proud to have been a part of this process of awakening.

Serena rekindles in me the Buddhist idea of *sharing of merit*.

Idam te punna kammam-asavakkahaya vayam hotu.

May our meritorious actions lead to the removal of all unwholesomeness.

– Leonard Levine

Chapter Three

The New Dentistry
Light Years Beyond Drill and Fill

By Farid Shodjaee, BSc, DDS

About Farid Shodjaee

A graduate of the McGill University School of Dentistry in Montreal, Dr. Farid Shodjaee holds a private general dental practice in Ottawa, Ontario, Canada.

Dr. Shodjaee enthusiastically travels to various centres around the world to further his knowledge of the latest concepts and techniques in his field.

Gentle of hand and light of spirit, Dr. Shodjaee has achieved remarkable results with his patients.

He places special emphasis in Biological Dentistry, Functional Jaw Orthopedics, Orthodontics, Craniomandibular Dysfunction and Tempromandibular Dysfunction.

Dr. Shodjaee lives happily in Chelsea, Quebec with his wife Laurie and their three sons.

Dr. Farid Shodjaee can be reached at:
The St. Laurent Dental Centre, 1200 St. Laurent Blvd.
Box 203, Ottawa, ON, K1K 3B8
613-744-6611 Ext. 241; Fax 613-744-5848
farid@drfarid.com
www.drfarid.com

THE NEW DENTISTRY
LIGHT YEARS BEYOND DRILL AND FILL

*Sickness reveals a lack of balance in the
human organism, an absence of equilibrium
in the forces essential for the normal
functioning of the human body.*

– Baha'i writings

A CASE STUDY

M.J., a 42-year-old woman, has not slept soundly for the past 25 years. She has been suffering from tension headaches, migraines, stiff neck muscles and sore teeth. She also becomes dizzy, feels nauseated and experiences blurry vision with pain around or behind her eyes. She experiences headaches in both right and left temple areas and in the back of her head. She grinds her teeth at night and her jaws are sore and tired when she wakes up. She had a car accident 26 years ago during which she sustained severe blows to her head and jaw and a whiplash injury to her neck. Every day upon awaking she takes numerous Advil pills for the pain. Although M.J. has seen many physicians and specialists for these health issues, sadly, no treatment has helped her so far.

I saw M.J. in February 2003 and did a complete assessment of her condition. I diagnosed her as having what we call Craniomandibular dysfunction, more commonly known as Tempromandibular joint (TMJ) dysfunction (TMD). The relationship of her lower jaw to her skull is not in a healthy position, thus reducing her adaptive capability range. She cannot open her mouth, bite or chew properly. When she goes through the normal daily functions of biting and chewing her food or even speaking, undue stress is placed on the numerous muscles throughout her face, head, jaw and neck. Adding this to the normal physical, mental and emotional stresses of life has put her over the edge to develop all the above symptoms.

Within a month of treatment, which painlessly and effortlessly established a more healthy position of her jaw in relation to her skull, some cranio-osteopathy treatment and some nutritional support, M.J. is free of her symptoms. In her own words: "Within days after treatment I noticed positive results. I sleep like a baby and wake up with no headaches or migraines. My jaw is not sore and I do not experience as much anxiety. I have not taken a single Advil for pain. On top of that I feel more energetic."

M.J. is not alone. It has been estimated that more that 50 million people in North America suffer from headaches. These headaches can be so debilitating that they can adversely affect people's ability to work and their relationship with family and friends. Although there can be many reasons for headaches, indeed many headache patients suffer from TMD.

The irony in M.J.'s story is that as a dentist I was never taught how to treat patients who had chronic pain due to TMD, and for years I told my patients that there was nothing I could do about their clicking jaw. Even worse, to my shame, I had no knowledge of any relationship that could exist between jaw joints and headaches or shoulder aches or even lower backaches. (Later I will explain in detail the Cranial-Dental-Sacral complex; that is, how the head, jaw and back are all connected to one another.)

15 YEARS EARLIER

I had just graduated from dental school at McGill University, which is rated as one of the best dental schools in Canada. I was very proud of my performance, having graduated fourth in my class in 1987. My wife Laurie and I were encouraged by her father to explore the grand north of Canada, where he had traveled for his work as an architect specializing in Northern housing. He suggested that I might find a position as a town dentist.

Through the Regie de l'assurance maladie (Quebec Medical Health Plan), I secured a job in the small town of Fort Rupert in James Bay, Quebec. So as soon as we both graduated from McGill (Laurie got an MA in political science), we were off to James Bay.

For the next two years I worked as a dentist in this little town of 1400 people. I was busy from nine a.m. to five p.m. from the day I arrived until we left. The experience of just doing basic dentistry was great and having the tranquility of the North after living in Montreal for eight years, although I do love Montreal, was comforting. My greatest impression of my work in the North, an impression that has stayed with me over the years, is how the white man's diet has ruined the Cree Indians' health, and especially their teeth. (Later I will point out specific research done by Dr. Weston Price in this area.)

After leaving Fort Rupert we came to the Ottawa area, which we thought would be a good place for me to set up a private dental practice and for Laurie to start her career in her chosen field of study, but life events took us in a new direction. We were introduced through friends and family to homeopathy. The big event that turned us completely toward exploring a different health-care system for our family was when my second son, after receiving the usual childhood PPD vaccination, showed a severe reaction that resulted in seizures. Miraculously, this reaction ceased immediately when treated with homeopathy. We were both astounded and greatly relieved.

In our search to find a health-care system for our family, I learned that what we refer to as health care these days is very confusing. Dr. Robert Walker, an Australian chiropractor, divides our present health-care system into three levels:[1]

1. Crises care: emergency care at the hospital level to prevent loss of life.

---

1 Walker, Dr. Robert, *Chirodontics the Logic of Health*, www.chirodontics.com

2. Symptom care: eliminating patients' symptoms (the primary role of most physicians and today's health-care system in general).

3. Health care: creating optimal, asymptomatic health.

When we realized the symptom focus rather than health focus of our current health-care system, our family chose to move to homeopathy, and Laurie began her studies as a homeopathic practitioner. Meanwhile I had this busy thriving and growing dental practice in Ottawa in a group partnership with some of Ottawa's best at the St. Laurent Dental Centre.

Somehow, perhaps because of my upbringing, I have come to love and enjoy learning new things. So, for many years I have been exploring different areas of dentistry, taking a wide variety of courses, and learning new procedures and techniques. I was so involved in the excitement of my learning that it took me about ten years to realize that dentistry should be more than drill and fill. Perhaps you, like me, are wondering why it took me so long.

One of the health areas in which I was doing a lot of reading was mind-body medicine. Today, in all areas of medicine including dentistry, students are taught how systems work by tearing the body apart and studying bits and pieces of the body at a time. They never look at the patient as a whole. Worse, when we doctors or dentists choose to specialize, we work so deeply in a single area of specialty that we can forget this area's connection to the rest of the body, and that it all works as a whole. A good friend of mine who is an ophthalmologist remarked that we are dissecting the human body into such small areas and offering so many subspecialties that soon our greatest specialists know everything about nothing. He had a great teacher who, every once in a while, would grab his collar, pull him back from a patient and ask him to look at the whole picture.

In my research and reading in the field of dentistry and how it relates to the whole body as part of a unique system, I learned about Biological Dentistry. One of its aspects, the Cranial Dental Sacral Complex, has become my work's passion. Unfortunately, since this aspect of dentistry is the least understood, little of it is taught in North American dental schools. Indeed, very few professors of dentistry have ever had any training in this area. Luckily, after much research through the American Wholistic Dental Association, I have been able to find practitioners who not only excel in this area but also provide teaching for other interested dentists. I was on my way.

Now, let me introduce you to the concept of Biological Dentistry and a variety of areas that biological dentists are working on today to provide a more wholistic approach to what used to be only "drill and fill."

BIOLOGICAL DENTISTRY

A better name for Biological Dentistry is Dentistry with Consciousness. I remember when I was a dental student there was a sign posted in the office window of one of my teachers. It read, "I am not a drill and fill doctor." He was ahead of his time.

As humanity is evolving, so are our approaches in dental health. As the 21st century is upon us, a new era of dentistry is coming of age, an era that combines a sophisticated mechanical approach with more evolved biological or pro-biotic (life-supporting) system of dental medicine. It is like a marriage between high-tech dentistry and ancient wisdom that acknowledges and respects the health of the entire body. Below are five areas that biological dentistry is focusing on, followed by a short explanation of each area:

1. Dental material biocompatibility
2. Focal oral infection (from root canalled teeth, extraction sites and gum diseased teeth)
3. Energy disturbances to the body (galvanic shock)
4. Influence of nutrition on oral health
5. Cranial, dental, sacral complex

Dental Material Biocompatibility

The topic that has dominated this area is the use of mercury in amalgam fillings. The unfortunate position of organized dentistry and the misstated biocompatibility of this material are well known by many readers. I will refer to only two books in this area. Dr. Hal Huggins in *It's All in Your Head, The Link Between Mercury Amalgam and Illness*[2] clearly states the dangerous effect of mercury in dental amalgams in the following 5 categories:

1. Neurological (motor and sensory) e.g.: seizures and MS

2. Immunological e.g.: Lupus, arthritis

3. Cardiovascular e.g.: blood pressure, tachycardia

4. Collagen: e.g.: Osteoarthritis

5. Miscellaneous e.g.: chronic fatigue, digestion problem, brain fog, etc.

The other book, by Quicksilver Associates, is entitled *The Mercury in Your Mouth: The Truth About "Silver" Dental Fillings*.[3] Both books were written in order to provide the general public with valuable information of which even your dentist may not be aware.

Other potentially toxic dental materials in question include nickel, which has been used in partial dentures and crowns. The dissociation of this metal and migration to and absorption in other parts of the body can cause malfunctioning of other systems such as the immune system. Evaluating the replacing of lost teeth should include consideration of the biocompatibility of the materials to be used. In addition to being a known carcinogen, nickel also interferes with the body's electromagnetic field.

Most conventional root canal treatment also employs a variety of products that are very harmful and caustic to the surrounding tissue. The biocompatibility of the dental materials to be employed can be assessed by one of the following methods:

1. Serum testing by antigen-antibody precipitation test

2. Electrodermal testing

3. Applied Kinesiology muscle testing

2   Huggins, Dr. Hal A, *It's All in Your head: The Link Between Mercury Amalgam and Illness*, Avery Publishing, 1993.

3   Quicksilver Associates, *The Mercury in Your Mouth*, Quicksilver Press, 1998.

One last thing to consider before calling a product completely safe is to ensure that it is compatible with our body frequency. This can be done by bioenergetic assessment or cranial evaluation in contact with the material. A competent, well-trained dentist can do this for you.

Focal Oral Infection

There are hidden or residual infection areas that are called dental interference fields or foci. The main source of these hidden fields are either the asymptomatic residual infections of teeth with root canal as discussed by Dr. George E. Meinig in *Root Canal Cover-up*[4] or the extraction site of the teeth known as jaw cavitations as described by Susan Stockton in *Beyond Amalgam: the hidden health hazard posed by jawbone cavitations.*[5] The bacteria active in these residual infection fields can migrate and cause degenerative diseases in other parts of the human body.

The pioneer in this field was Dr. Weston Price whose research dates back to the 1930s. Studies have shown that up to 75 percent of root canalled teeth that have no symptoms have residual bacterial infection in their dentinal tubules.[4,6]

Energy Disturbances to the Body

A phenomenon that is unfortunately often ignored in dentistry is how saliva can act as an electrolyte when dissimilar metals have been used in the mouth. This is exactly how a battery works. In the mouth it is called oral galvanism. The energy or electrical current generated by oral galvanism can cause disturbances in body organic function, membrane permeability, and can even initiate degenerative changes. The metallic energy can block the acupuncture meridian circuits associated with certain teeth, causing dysfunction in the respective organs. More about this can be found in the entitled Teeth to Body Chart on the

---

4   Meinig, George E. DDS. FACD, Root Canal Cover-up, BION Publishing, 2000.

5   Stockton, Susan, *Beyond Amalgam: The Hidden Health Hazard Posed by Jawbone Cavitations,* Power of One Publishing, 2001.

6   Price, Weston A., *Dental Infection and the Degenerative Diseases,* Penton Publishing, 1923.

---

website of Dr. Bill Wolfe.[7] He has a wonderful acupuncture meridian chart which shows the relationship between teeth and other areas of the body.

Influence of Nutrition on Oral Health

In the 1920s and '30s, Dr. Weston Price traveled around the world and studied many primitive populations. Those groups that followed their traditional nature-based diets enjoyed good health and vigour and those that turned to the "civilized" diet of processed, sugar-laden foods soon developed a variety of degenerative illnesses. They also displayed bad bites, narrow, crowded arches and tooth decay.[8]

Unfortunately, Dr. Weston's advice has been virtually disregarded. It would seem that one is never given a Nobel prize by finding out that the solution to many degenerative illnesses is as simple as eating the right, locally grown food. I guess it does not make as much financial sense as selling people something processed by big industries far away.

The Cranial, Dental, Sacral Complex

Sickness reveals a lack of equilibrium
in the forces essential for the normal functioning
of the human body.
– Baha'i Writings

This area of Biological Dentistry deals with the structural balance that influences our neurological, mental, emotional and physiological health. The Cranial, Dental, Sacral Complex is composed of our cranium, dental arches and teeth, spinal column and sacrum area.

Imagine our skeletal system as our skull held over our shoulder girdle by the neck and our spine positioned over our pelvic girdle. In other words, the human skeletal

---

7   Wolfe, Bill, D.D.S., N.M.D., *Teeth to Body Chart*, http://www.drwolfe.com/html/teeth-chart.html.

8   Price, Weston A., D.D.S., *Nutrition and Physical Degeneration*, Price-Pottenger Nutrition Foundation, 2000.

body consists of a spinal column with the head bone at one end and the tailbone at the other. Like all the other structures, balance is the key in stability. Dr. James Carlson observed that parallel relationships exist in the structurally stable human body[9] (figure 1) which permit it to maintain balance. These parallel planes include the ear plane, eye plane, shoulder plane, elbow and knee planes and pelvic plane. Dr. Carlson's observation revealed that the upper jaw or maxillae was another anatomic part that was also parallel to these other planes.

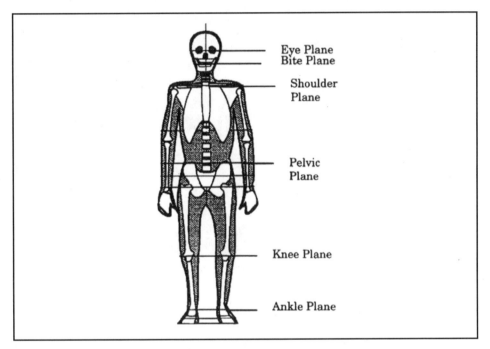

Eye Plane
Bite Plane

Shoulder Plane

Pelvic Plane

Knee Plane

Ankle Plane

Figure 1: The Parallel Planes of the Body

All the bones of the skull are connected not only through joints and/or sutures but also by muscles and the dural sheath (also known as the dural tube, dural membrane or meningeal membrane).

The dural tube (figure 2) is the tough, fibrous, thick, inelastic covering of the dura matter (brain). Its primary function is protection. This membrane, which is attached

9   Carlson, Dr. James, *Orthocranial Occlusion*, James Carlson Publishing, 2002.

to the inside of the cranium (figure 3), passes down to the spinal column, attaches to the first three cervical vertebrae, then travels down to the sacrum and ends at the second sacral tubercle.

This dural tube provides a functional link in the entire system. Any movement, however minute, in one part of the system has a compensatory effect in other parts. To give you an example of this intimate connection, a baby that was delivered by forceps could have cranial distortion resulting in lower back pain at the level of sacro-iliac joint (SI joint) later in life.

Figure 2: The Dural Tube

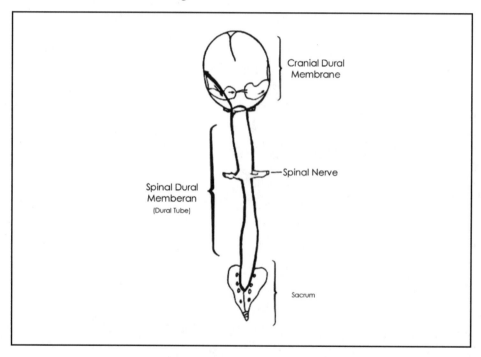

Figure 2. The dural tube is a continuous membrane that surrounds the brain, passes out of the base of the skull, attaches to the first three cervical vertebrae, and continues down the spinal cord where it finally attaches to the sacrum. This tube is the source for structural disturbances being transmitted from one part of the body to another. Because the body works reciprocally, imbalances in the skull can influence the neck, lower back, and pelvis and the reverse is also true.

(Courtesy of Dr. Gerald Smith)[10]

10   Smith, Dr. Gerald, *Headaches are not Forever*, ICNR Publishing, 1986.

Figure 3: The Cranial Dural Membranes

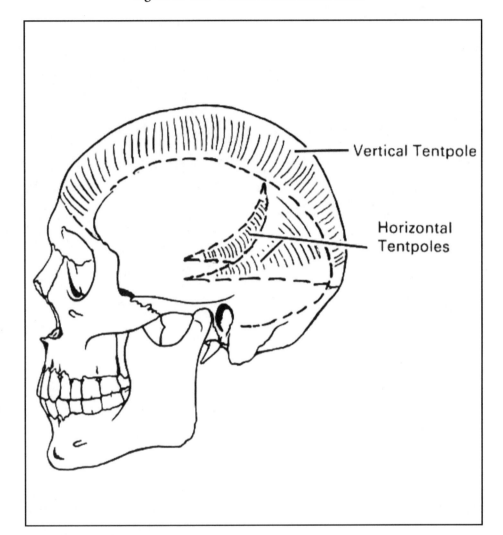

Vertical Tentpole

Horizontal Tentpoles

Figure 3: The cranial dural membranes act as stabilizers to the vault bones. Physical trauma (whiplash injuries, blows to the head, forceful tooth extraction, etc.) and dental malocclusions have the potential to disrupt dural membrane balance and normal cranial rhythm. Such changes can cause adverse neurological function throughout the body.

(Courtesy of Dr Gerald Smith)[11]

Closer to home for me, the upper teeth are set in the maxilla. The maxilla is not just a jaw, it represents the front third of the cranial base. If the upper jaw is distorted (crooked teeth, crossed bite, one side higher than the other, canted maxilla, etc.), then the forces generated by the unmatched biting teeth can distort the skull. To make things even more complicated, in the head and neck region there are 136 muscles. Muscle tension or spasm can influence cranial motion. Among these muscles are the muscles of mastication (chewing). Since these muscles are all attached to the skull, improper bite can often trigger muscle spasms, which in turn can jam the sutures and distort the cranial bones.

As if this were not enough, dental malocclusion (bad bite) like deep bite, cross bite (front or back), a constricted narrow upper arch, faulty crowns or dentures, high cant of maxilla, or under-developed lower jaw can all contribute to cranial distortion. Please read on to find out why this is so important.

CRANIAL MOTION

The combination of the elements in the body of man is more perfect
than the composition of any other being; it is mingled in absolute equilibrium,
therefore it is nobler and more perfect.

– Baha'i Writings

In 1939, Osteopath William Sutherland discovered that there is a rhythmic motion to our cranium. The adult cranium (figure 4) is composed of 28 bones. These bones are attached together at junctions called sutures. In the past, sutures were considered immovable joints, however the work of Dr. John Upledger proved that these sutures were viable structures[12] (figure 5).

---

12 Upledger, John and Do Retzlaff, Earnest W., "Diagnosis and treatment of Temporo-parietal suture head pain," *Osteopathic Medicine*, July 1978, pp. 19-26.

Figure 4: The Adult Cranium

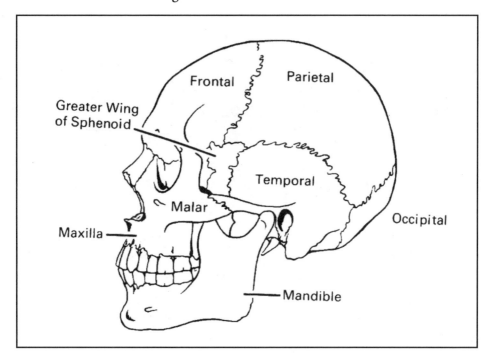

Figure 4. The cranium is a dynamic structure that is in a constant state of micro-motion. This motion can occur because of the inherent flexibility of bones plus the presence of the expansion joints or sutures that lie between each bone. Architects design buildings, bridges and roads with specific leeway for expansion, contraction and torsion. Nature likewise provides for similar allowances in the flexibility of its hard and soft tissues and their interconnections.

(Courtesy of Dr. Gerald Smith)[13]

The origin of cranial motion is thought to be the brain cells, so just as the lungs rhythmically contract and expand through breathing, so does our cranium. This cranial motion is also known as Primary Respiratory Mechanism (PRM).[14] PRM is independent of all other body rhythms like heartbeat, breathing, and the waves of movement that pass food along the intestines.

---

13 Smith, Dr. Gerald, ibid.

14 Sneddon, Peta and Cosechi, Paolo, *Discover Osteopathy*, Ulysses Press, 1997.

Figure 5: Dural Membrane and Suture Relationship

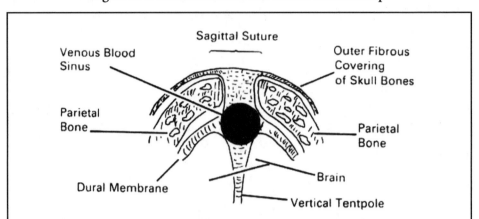

Figure 5. Scientists have documented the existence of nerves, blood vessels and connecting fibres in the sutural areas. Anatomists have also shown the direct physical connection between the inside and outside of the skull. The dural membrane that surrounds the brain communicates with and influences the outside of the skull by means of an outer fibrous layer. This layer passes through the sutures and covers the bony portions of the skull. For this reason, internal tension has the potential to cause external changes such as muscle spasm (a migraine patient's scalp can become sore from simple brushing) and vice-type pressure. The reverse is also true. Whether the headache is due to physical tension or a vascular migraine, the dural membrane will be affected.

(Courtesy of Dr. Gerald Smith)[15]

PRM is felt as the expansion and contraction of the head and body. The mechanism is characterized by the light movement of the bones of the skull and the sacrum, the dural tube and the central nervous system with the flow of cerebrospinal fluid (CSF) (figure 6). Sutherland did experiments on himself by restricting various bones of his head. He experienced both adverse physiological changes throughout his body and unpleasant emotions. He then concluded that good physiological and mental health depends not only on the bones of the cranium being in the right position, but also on the ability of the sutures to allow this micro-motion to happen.

---

15 Smith, Dr. Gerald, *Headaches Are Not Forever*, ibid.

Figure 6: The Cerebrospinal Fluid

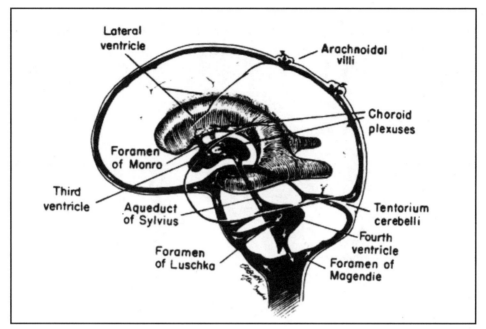

Figure 6. The cerebrospinal fluid (CSF) is produced by choroid plexuses within the ventricles of the brain. Increased production occurs with increased stimulation of the parasympathetic (PNS) part of the nervous system. The PNS is located primarily in the cranium and sacral part of the body. Distortions of the skull bones or pelvic area have the potential to cause an increased quantity of CSF and raise intracranial pressure.

(Courtesy of Gerald Smith)[16]

This cranial motion can further be divided into two basic micro-motions: primary and secondary. Primary micro-motion involves the independent movement of the skull and spinal cord, which facilitates the movement of CSF, articular motion of the cranial bones and involuntary motion of the sacrum. Secondary cranial respiratory motion synchronizes with our breathing cycles of inhalation and exhalation. Inhalation expands the cranium while exhalation reduces it.

16 ibid.

Both primary and secondary respiration is coordinated by the dural tube. This tube is the source of structural disturbances transmitted from one part of the spinal column (sacrum) to the other (skull). Because our skeletal system works reciprocally, any imbalance in the cranium can affect the neck, lower back, pelvis and vice versa (figure 7.)

Figure 7: The Body as a Slinky

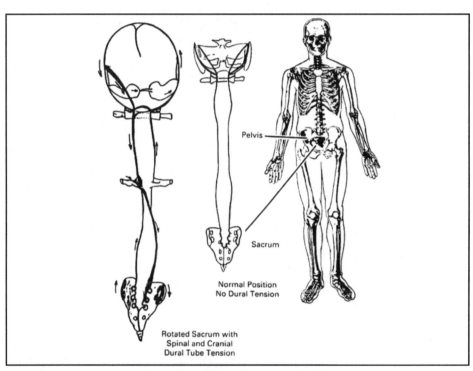

Figure 7. In reality, the body functions just like a slinky. A distortion at one end will be reflected to its area compensation. For example, the bones of the hands and feet work reciprocally as well as the ankle and wrist, knee and elbow, pelvis and shoulders. One of the main connecting links of the body that enables this slinky effect to occur is the dural tube. Joint receptors and neuromuscular biofeedback provide other means by which the body functions reciprocally.

(Courtesy of Gerald Smith)[17]

17 ibid.

I hope it has become clear that imbalances in any part of this system can interfere with cranial motion and cause disease in our system. Physical traumas such as whiplash injury to the neck or pelvis trauma from falling off a horse, bad posture caused by working in front of computer extensively, and dental problems such as bad bite are examples of things that can disturb the balance in the system. These can cause cranial distortion and restrict cranial motion eliciting clinical symptoms such as headache, dizziness, numbness, muscle spasm, faulty digestion, jaw pain, irregular heart beat, tinnitus (figure 10), migraines (figure 8), circulatory problems, chronic fatigue, sinusitis, constipation, neck ache, shoulder ache, eye pain and facial pain.

Figure 8: The Dural Tube and its Role in Migraine

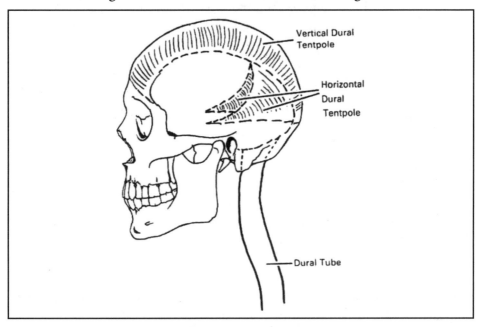

Figure 8: Migraine headaches usually affect one-half of the victim's head. Since the dural tube is a reciprocating membrane, tension or torquing in the skull will cause one side to be in traction while the other side provides the slack. The nerves passing through the tensioned side will be responsible for the varied and extensive pains. The dural torquing can result from a single or various combinations of structural distortion involving the pelvis, spinal vertebrae, dental malocclusion or cranial bone restrictions. These structural problems can be triggered by emotional, physical, nutritional or physiological stressors (e.g. organ dysfunction, under-active thyroid, muscle spasm or weakness, and fixed and removable dental bridgework)

(Courtesy of Dr. Gerald Smith)[18]

18 ibid.

Closer to my area of expertise, patients with a deep overbite, underdeveloped lower jaw, cross bite, or collapsed bite may experience cranial distortion and dural torque. Many of them suffer from headaches, migraines, neck and shoulder stiffness and lower back pain. Some may have itchiness or stuffiness in the ears and many have clicking jaw joints.

Among the other dental conditions is conventional orthodontics that involved the amputation of premolar teeth to mechanically achieve esthetic arches by moving back the upper six front teeth. This caused restriction of the maxilla, palatine, vomer and sphenoid skull bones and contributed further to an already forward head position and loss of normal curvature of the cervical vertebra. Studies have shown that patients with the above treatment have a limited neck movement and compressed upper cervical vertebra especially at the level of C1 to C3. They are already at a disadvantage with regard to their dental, cervical and cranial balance. If these individuals are involved in an accident and experience a whiplash injury to their neck, they will never fully recover unless their structural imbalance is addressed.

WHOLISTIC DENTAL/MEDICAL EVALUATION

Dr. Gerald Smith of Langhorne, Pennsylvania (my teacher and mentor in this field), over 20 years ago pioneered a very thorough and wholistic approach to patient evaluation which he named Physiological Adaptive Range (PAR).

Dr. Smith is a dentist, class of 1969 from Temple University School of dentistry. He further went on to postgraduate studies in Osteopathics, Dental Orthopedics, Orthodontics, Nutrition and Physical Therapy. I have read all of his written material and have received one-on-one hands-on training at his office. In Dr. Smith's own words:

The PAR concept is based on the fact that all physiological structures (bones, ligaments, muscles, membranes, organs, nervous system, etc.) and processes (digestion, detoxification, blood formation, tissue repair, etc.) and fluids (enzymes, saliva, hormones, blood, lymph, perspiration, etc.) function within adaptable ranges. .... The body has the ability to compensate and maintain a state of equilibrium within its genetic boundaries. Deviation

---

19 Smith, Dr. Gerald H., *Cranial-Dental-Sacral Complex: A Physiological Concept and a Common Sense Approach to TMJ Therapy*, ICNR Publishing, 1983.

beyond these physiological adaptive ranges disrupts the body's homeostasis and shifts function into a state of imbalance.[19]

> *The outer, physical causal factor in disease is a disturbance in the balance, the proportionate equilibrium of all those elements of which the human body is composed.*
>
> – Baha'i Writings

Dr. Smith has divided his PAR exam into the following areas

1. Cranial Evaluation

2. Dental Evaluation

3. Pelvic Evaluation

4. Physiological and Nutritional Evaluation

5. Psychological and Emotional Evaluation

The first three areas of the structural evaluation are intimately connected to our nervous system. The physiological evaluation assesses all our organs and physiological processes, and the nutritional evaluation determines our deficiencies and what we need to take to supplement our organs and processes to optimal health. Last, but not least, our psychological and emotional health is evaluated because it has an overwhelming effect on our physiology. This is where the origins of disease come from and what happens to our physical body is really the mechanics of the disease. I use the above evaluation to assess my patients, especially those who are suffering from chronic pain. As you have most likely already guessed, the treatment is to return the patient to within their adaptive range capability.

This is an integrated treatment technique and it requires a multidisciplinary approach. I work closely with a group of fine wholistic practitioners including a cranial osteopath, chiropractor, homeopath and physical therapist, some of whom are contributors to this book. We strive to bring our patients to optimal health, not to just mask symptoms.

BACK TO M.J.

I would like to return to patient M.J.'s story that began this chapter in order to give you an idea of how we used this integrated treatment technique for her.

M.J. was referred to my office by one of my colleagues for suspicion of Tempromandibular Dysfunction (TMD) because of the symptoms she was experiencing.

My PAR examination revealed the following:

1. Cranial complex: Overall in good health except some structural/bone distortion in temple areas, and cranial rhythm and amplitude worsen when patient puts her teeth together.

2. Dental complex: Heavily restored dentition, many root canalled teeth. Underdeveloped lower jaw and collapsed deep bite.

3. Physiological, nutrition complex: Compressed cervical vertebrae (whiplash injury 20 years ago), sore neck and shoulder muscles, weak adrenal and thyroid glands and over-stimulated autonomic nervous system.

4. Psychological, emotional complex: In spite of her challenges in life she is strong and optimistic, but overall under lots of stress.

M.J. was diagnosed as dental major with compensatory cranial and cervical distortion and physiological disturbances, all exacerbated with whiplash injury.

Our integrated treatment technique included the following:

a. Repositioning or realignment of the lower jaw to her skull with a temporary dental appliance.

b. Cranial-Sacral osteopathy treatment for proper cranial, cervical and pelvic health.

c. Nutritional support for repairs and healing of muscle tissue and supporting of her glandular function through natural vitamins and supplements.[20]

d. Homeopathic care for physiological and/or psychological balance.

Within days, as quoted earlier, her symptoms were gone and she was brought back to within her physiological adaptive range. She is healthy at this point and

20 Wolocott, William and Fahey, Trish, *The Metabolic Typing Diet*, Broadway Books, 2002.

enjoying a life free from migraines and sore muscles and wakes up in the morning refreshed rather than with head, jaw and teeth aches.

AUTONOMIC NERVOUS SYSTEM (ANS) CONSIDERATIONS IN CRANIOMANDIBULAR DYSFUNCTION (CMD)

Before I get into the negative effects of dural torque on ANS, I would like to provide some background information about ANS.

ANS consists of the sensory and motor nervous system that runs between the central nervous system (CNS) and various internal organs such as the heart, lungs, viscera and glands. ANS is responsible for monitoring conditions in the internal environment and bringing about appropriate changes in them. The contraction of smooth muscle and cardiac muscle is controlled by motor neurons of the ANS. The action of ANS is largely involuntary. The ANS has two subdivisions, the sympathetic and parasympathetic nervous systems.

Both of these systems act to regulate the function of ANS, much like the gas pedal and brake in your car. One system stimulates, the other inhibits functions of the affected organ (figure 9). For example, the sympathetic system output does the following:

- Stimulates heartbeat

- Raises blood pressure

- Dilates pupils, trachea, bronchi

- Stimulates conversion of glycogen into glucose in liver

- Shunts blood away from skin and viscera to skeletal muscles, brain and heart

- Inhibits peristalsis in gastrointestinal tract

- Inhibits contraction of bladder and rectum

- Inhibits salivary flow

In short, stimulation of the sympathetic branch of the ANS prepares the body for emergencies, the "fight or flight" response, one of the most primary animalistic response left in humans.

PARASYMPATHETIC STIMULATION CAUSES:

- Slowing of heartbeat
- Lowering of blood pressure
- Contraction of pupils
- Increased blood flow to skin and viscera
- Peristalsis of GI tract

In short, the parasympathetic system returns the body functions to normal after they have been altered by sympathetic stimulation. Although the ANS is considered to be involuntary, this is not entirely true. A certain amount of conscious control can be exerted over the system. For example, meditation can alter a number of autonomic functions involving heart rate, rate of oxygen consumption, blood pressure, etc.

Figure 9: The Autonomic Nervous System

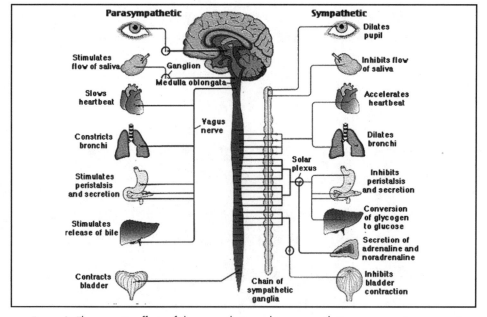

Figure 9: The opposite effects of the sympathetic and parasympathetic nervous systems on various organs.

ANATOMICAL CONSIDERATIONS OF ANS[21]

The ANS is located in the brain stem. The brain stem is situated outside the skull at the level of upper cervical area (figure 10).

Figure 10: The Upper Cervical Area

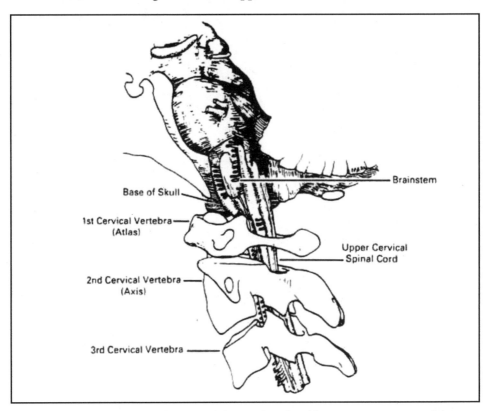

Figure 10. The upper cervical portion of the spinal cord and brainstem represent one of the most important areas of the nervous system. Within this area lie the autonomic life sustaining centres-heartbeat, respiration, consciousness and blood pressure. Also present are centres that control motor and sensory function to and from the face, eyes, mouth and throat.

Distortion of the dural tube in this vital region has the potential to disrupt cerebrospinal fluid and blood flow to these important centres. Singly or in combination, the effects of vertebrae subluxations (malposition), muscle spasm (due to tension or whiplash injury), dural tension from a rotated pelvis or a dental malocclusion will have far-reaching motor and sensory disturbances throughout the body.

(Courtesy of Gerald Smith)[22]

21 Smith, Dr. Gerald H., *Alternative Treatment for Conquering Chronic Pain*, ICNR Publishing, 1998.

22 http://users.rcn.com/jkimball.ma.ultranet/BiologyPages/P/PNS.html#CranialNerves.

Any structural disturbances in this area can upset the very essential balance or homeostasis of the ANS. If this area of the ANS is structurally compromised, it can have far-reaching motor and sensory disturbances throughout the body. As discussed earlier, the ANS is the life sustaining centre for heartbeat, respiration, consciousness, blood pressure, cerebrospinal fluid (CSF) regulation, and motor and sensory function to and from the face, eyes, mouth and throat just to mention few.

The following conditions can structurally influence the upper cervical area and disturb ANS function:

1. Vertebral subluxation (malposition)

2. Muscle spasm due to tension or whiplash injury

3. Dural tension or torque (from rotated pelvic or SI joint, bad bite, cranial distortion)

(Note that the dural tube attaches to the upper 3 cervical vertebrae.)

THE MANDIBULAR POSITION IN CMD

To complicate CMD further, the centre of the rotation of the lower jaw is at the second cervical vertebrae. It has been proven that a collapsed bite and/or retruded lower jaw will also cause upper cervical compression and can influence the ANS.

THE TEMPORAL BONES' ROLE IN CMD

Another key anatomical factor that can have a major role in Craniomandibular dysfunction (CMD) are the temporal bones (figure 4). Two rather large bones on either side of the skull that house the condyles of the mandible and ears. The following features of the temporal bones affect CMD:

1. Two primary muscles of mastication, masseter and temporalis, attach to the temporal bones.

2. The temporal bones articulate with occipital, parietals, and sphenoid, zygoma and mandibular condyles (figure 4).

3. The temporal bones function in a synchronous arrangement with the ileum of the pelvis due to the dural tube interrelationship (figure 7).

4. The dural tube is attached to internal aspect of temporal bone via a horizontal tent pole called tentorium cerebelli (figure 3). Passing between the leaves of this fibrous attachment are the cranial nerves III, IV, V, VI, (nerves to all eye muscles.) Actually, nine out of 12 cranial nerves are in close relationship or proximity to the temporal bones. (CN III through XI)

5. Some neck muscles such as the sternocleidomastoid, digasteric and capitis muscles are attached to temporal bones.

The following are some common symptoms of temporal bone distortion (figure 11):

- Conductive hearing loss

- Disequilibrium (vertigo)

- Head pain

- Vagatonia (increased vaga activity)

- Motor eye dysfunction

- Dyslexia

- Recurrent arm and shoulder pain

In essence, the temporal bones are the keystone of the cranium and the following factors can cause temporal bone distortion:

1. Chronic dental malocclusion: bad bite, cross bite, underdeveloped lower jaw, collapsed bite, malpositioned mandibular condyles

2. Muscle spasm associated with the temporal bones; for example masseter, temporalis, sternocliedomastoid, digasteric, etc.

3. Dural torque (of any origin)

4. Compensation for positional changes of ileum

5. Sutural distortion with other cranial bones, mainly sphenoid, occipital and parietals

Figure 11: TMJ and Ear Connection

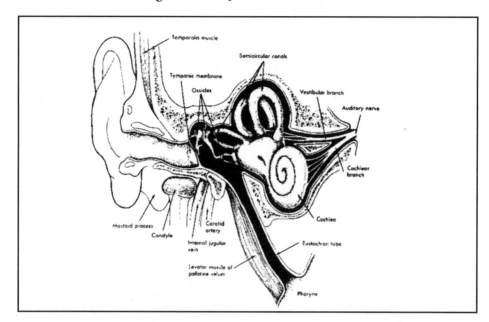

The jaw joint lies in close proximity to the middle ear. Distortions of jaw position due to an improper bite, muscle spasm, or a retrusion of the jaw resulting from a whiplash injury have the potential to cause ear problems such as ear noises — ringing, hissing, buzzing, conductive hearing loss, increased pressure and pain. They can also affect our balance mechanism.

(Courtesy of Dr. Gerald Smith)[23]

Once anatomical distortion of the various kinds mentioned above exceeds the body's physiological adaptive capability, the body will show the symptoms of disease. I have already mentioned many symptoms associated with the temporal bones. The following symptoms can be experienced due to ANS disturbances. Note how similar these symptoms are to those of migraines:

- Sympathetic dominance: Blockage of nasal sinuses, eye sensitivity to light

- Parasympathetic dominance: Nausea, vomiting, diarrhea and abdominal pains

Structurally, the cranium and sacrum provide parasympathetic stimulation and the thoraco-lumbar area of the spine provides sympathetic activity. The above symptoms of migraines are due to ANS imbalances.

---

23   Smith, Dr. Gerald, *Headaches Are Not Forever*, ibid.

If we consider the above symptoms and those due to temporal bone distortion such as disequilibrium, dizziness, ringing and stuffiness in the ears, and visual disturbances associated with distortion of sphenoid bone, then we have all the symptoms of classic migraine that such a large percentage of the population suffer from, and spend millions of dollars to treat with medication.

All but two of the eye muscles are attached to the lesser wing of the sphenoid, so any cranial lesion affecting the sphenoid bone like that of a canted maxilla can distort the eye muscles and create visual disturbances. Another cause of visual disturbance can be distorted temporal bones that affect the eye nerve supply (CN III, IV, V, VI associated with the temporal bones innervate the eye).

To successfully treat migraine sufferers one must assess the patient in all the areas of Physiological Adaptive Range (PAR) and correct all the imbalances, whether the disturbances may be physiological, nutritional, psychological, emotional or skeletal. It is nonsense to give these patient drugs and hope for the best.

In my practice, I rely on a combination of treatments. I recommend homeopathy to correct physiological and/or psychological imbalances. I recommend nutritional support and the Metabolic Typing Diet (Wolocott [24]) to treat nutritional imbalances. I advocate cranial osteopathy for proper skeletal balance, and of course, I offer biological dentistry for optimal health.

SOME THOUGHTS ON CLOSING

Finally, the perfection of each individual being, that is to say
the perfection which you now see in man or apart from him,
with regard to their atoms, members, or powers,
is due to the composition of the elements, to their measure,
to their balance, to the mode of their combination,
and to mutual influence. When all these are gathered together,
then man exists.

– Baha'i Writings

24 | Wolocott, William and Fahey, Trish, *The Metabolic Typing Diet*, Broadway Books, 2002.

Our current science is drawn from the infancy of humanity and as humanity comes of age with some pain and discomfort, similar to a child that is going through puberty, our way of thinking will change. In the last 200 years, even though Newton was a great scientist, his influence and that of French philosopher Descartes have been so dominant in our culture that our whole culture and even our science has become the victim of what Dr. Deepak Chopra calls "superstition of materialism."

The superstition of materialism says that we believe we are material beings living in this material world. We have learned how to manufacture thoughts. We have thoughts, feelings, likes, dislikes and we fall in love all because of a dance of molecules. Consciousness, we are told, is a by-product of matter. This is the superstition.

Fortunately we are in the midst of what can only be called the climactic overthrow of the superstition of materialism and we are going through this because of our new science that is coming from a maturing humanity. We are realizing a new understanding of our reality through quantum physics and a new understanding of nature based on mechanism of perception.

Because of these two understandings, we now have evidence that our true nature is not matter at all, that we are actually composed of non-matter, that the building blocks of anything that we call stuff is actually non-stuff. The poets knew that long before our scientists, as William Blake says in his poem Auguries of Innocence:

To see a World in a Grain of Sand

And a Heaven in a Wild Flower

Hold Infinity in a palm of your hand

And Eternity in an hour

We are Led to Believe a Lie

When we see not Thro the Eye

Which was Born in a Night to perish in a Night

When the Soul Slept in the Beams of Light

I cannot overemphasize the principle of universal balance. There is a vedic (ancient Indian) saying that goes like this:

As is the atom so is the universe

As is the microcosm so is the macrocosm

As is the human body so is the cosmic body

As is the human mind so is the cosmic mind

When the universe functions based on this principle of balance, so should the human mind, body and soul. The Chinese knew this 5000 years ago through the concept of Ying and Yang. This balance exists in all areas of human life, whether physical, emotional, mental, social and spiritual.

I have explored ever so slightly this balance through the concept of PAR (Dr. Gerald Smith) as it relates mainly to our physicality. I also hope that I have clearly demonstrated that there is a profound and inseparable connection between the different physical aspects of our body. It is ludicrous to break down the human body into separate systems, study them individually, and treat them separately in times of illness. I have not even touched on life's emotional, mental, social and spiritual aspects, which could be as clearly demonstrated to be connected to our physicality and well-being, and even at times the root cause of disease.

Total health and well-being is a personal journey that one should consciously undertake. This journey, like traveling around the world, brings knowledge and understanding of humanity to our consciousness and prepares us further for the journey of life. As my teacher once said, "We are born naked in this world and leave with a suit on. The rest in between is fun and games."

Acknowledgements

I would like to thank and offer my gratitude:

To my family for a wonderful support in my quest to learn more in this limitless field of health.

To my patients for supporting me all these years to a better understanding of dental health and patient care.

To my homeopaths Patty Smith and Rudi Verspoor who have challenged me to explore wholistic dentistry.

To my teacher Dr. Gerald Smith for his way-out-in-left-field outlook on dentistry.

To my patient, editor, and friend Serena Williamson for her individual initiative to get this book off the ground and make my writings understandable.

To my staff who are very supportive of my bringing new challenges to our practice.

– Farid Shodjaee

Chapter Four

Stories from the Couch
Wholistic Psychotherapy and Healing

By Mary Rothschild, MSW, DHHP, HD(RHom)

Clinical social worker, certified psychoanalyst,
doctor of homeopathy

About Mary Rothschild

Mary Rothschild has a Masters of Social Work from Simmons Graduate School of Social Work (Boston, MA), a certificate in Psychoanalysis from The New York Center for Psychoanalytic Training (New York, NY), and was a training analyst, supervisor and teacher at The Chicago Center for Psychoanalytic Study (Chicago, IL).

She holds a DHHP from the Hahnemann Center for Heilkunst and Homeopathy (Ottawa, ON) and is a Doctor of Homeopathy. A practising psychotherapist for many years, Mary uses a variety of techniques to help people achieve the changes they want to make in their lives.

Born and raised in Chicago, Mary now lives in Manotick, Ontario with her two teenage daughters, two therapy dogs and two cats.

Mary Rothschild can be reached at:
613-692-6464
natrldoc@rogers.com.

STORIES FROM THE COUCH
WHOLISTIC PSYCHOTHERAPY AND HEALING

During my second year internship, one of my patients was a 50-year-old, chronic schizophrenic named George. No one else wanted his case, as he was never going to leave Boston State Mental Hospital. He shuffled instead of walked, always wore slippers, grey, food stained pants grabbed at random from the hospital laundry, a plaid shirt, a tweed jacket and a polka dot bow tie.

One night, a young man was admitted to the ward who thought he was Moses. The next day, George appeared wearing a yarmulke (skull cap) and told me he was a rabbi. When I told him he wasn't and that he was Catholic, he told me that he was indeed a rabbi and that Moses himself had told him so. I laughed and told him that I couldn't argue with an authority like that.

On my last day there, George took my hand, kissed it, and told me that I was his friend and he would miss me. I did the only thing I could do — I cried.

I often wonder what happened to George; I imagine he lived out the rest of his life there. I only hope someone else bought him the chocolate doughnuts he loved. George taught me the value of humour in therapy and that the client's perception of reality needs to be appreciated. Being right, even if it is to help the client see reality, is not always so important. He also taught me that it was alright to show my feelings. It seems odd to think there was a time that I didn't do that, but my training was to keep my feelings to myself, to not "contaminate" the therapy so the client's feelings can be analyzed without being tainted by what the therapist might feel.

HOW I BECAME WHO I AM

I was raised in a traditional, medical family. Even the therapists I saw were very traditional. The child psychiatrist I went to talked only when I did. If I remained silent, so did she. I still remember one very long session, when I was about nine, when we both sat in silence for the entire hour. It seemed unreasonable and inhumane to me then, and it still does all these years later.

After graduating with a degree in liberal arts, I went to the London School of Economics to do a master in economics. No social work school for me! I didn't want to do what other women were doing. Three weeks into my PhD program in economics in Boston, I walked into my advisor's office and told him that I didn't want to get out of bed in the morning because I hated what I was doing. He wisely told me that if I wasn't enjoying it, I should quit. I did — that same day.

Realizing that I missed working with people, I applied to a graduate program in clinical social work starting the next fall. Much as I loved my internships, my time there was spent regurgitating back what I was being taught. No one wanted to explore new techniques, the training was traditional, and even my analyst was very formal and distant, sitting so I couldn't see him.

Shortly after graduating and moving to New York, my marriage was disintegrating and I went back into therapy. I didn't know much about my therapist except that I could trust him, which was all I really needed to know. After a long time of getting nowhere and using free association to stay away from anything scary, he changed tactics and became more loving. (Only later did I learn that he presented my case at a conference entitled Working with your Most Difficult Client!) He utilized different techniques — role-playing, breathing, psychovisualizations, imaginary trips inside my body and more. He also shared information about himself when it was helpful for me. Of course, I had to analyze why I wanted to know and what it meant to me, but the openness was there. I learned that therapy is the place to learn what a loving, trusting relationship is, and that to do that, the therapist has to be genuine and loving. He even taught me how to hug after telling me that I hugged like the Cincinnati arch.

His openness and willingness to use a variety of techniques and even to create new ones changed who I became as a therapist. While I still practised as a psychoanalyst in those days (many of my clients came four or five times a week and lay on the couch — something that isn't done much anymore), I no longer used the traditional, impersonal approach I was originally taught. Interestingly, Freud, whose approach in which I was originally trained, was anything but impersonal.

I began to work with the whole person, and my view of what's included in this whole has evolved over time. It grew from believing that our experiences as a child influence what we experience as adults to include our life lessons, karma and past lives. I had always believed that each of us is unique and comes into the world with certain strengths and vulnerabilities that interact with our environment and relationships. Now I included karma, past life experiences and life lessons to be learned.

I have also long believed that the mind and body are intimately connected and profoundly affect each other. I remember going into a session one day with a scratchy, sore throat, and I was sure I was getting sick. After working on what I didn't want to say, my throat didn't hurt any longer and I felt fine. My body no longer needed to express what, until then, I wouldn't. Interestingly, I used to say the word "couldn't" but changed that as well. When we say that we cannot do something, it implies that there are physical limitations making the doing impossible. Saying I "wouldn't" or "chose not to" instead implies choice rather than impossibility and opens the door to examining the why not.)

SHARING MYSELF

One of the most important changes I made in my psychotherapeutic practice was to share my relevant life experiences with my clients. It is much easier to remain a blank screen because then you never have to examine if you want to tell your client something about yourself for his or her growth or for your own ends. Not everyone benefits from sharing, so another task is to know when to share and when not to. Sharing may be supportive, instructive, or something as basic as building a relationship.

Many years ago I was seeing a very bright, young women in analysis. (She was one of my two analytic clients when I did my analytic training.) She lived in a house with her parents, her sister, seven televisions and no meaningful conversations. Her family never discussed ideas, books, politics or the like. There was always a television on, and they sat and watched it in silence. We spent many sessions talking about movies, hairstyles, makeup, books, news items and anything else that interested her. I would also bring up subjects that I wanted to expose her to, and I shared my opinions and views. My supervisor in my postgraduate analytic training program told me that my client was merely being resistant to working therapeutically, and that she was wasting time. I'm certain of what else she would have said had she known that my analytic training client sat up rather than reclined on the couch during these sessions. I saw it differently because I was no longer traditional. Through our conversations, my client learned to relate, she had a role model very different than she was used to, and her intellectual horizons opened up. She developed new interests and began to form her own opinions about the world.

SELF-DISCLOSURE – OR HOW MUCH DO YOU WANT TO KNOW ABOUT ME?

Sharing personal information, which is part of sharing yourself, is a sticky and tricky issue for therapists. It needs to be in the best interests of the client — not just because the therapist needs to talk. There are many reasons for sharing, and there are also many reasons for not sharing, and the therapist has to be very clear about them.

I had a client whose mother had been so intrusive that she was afraid to trust anyone and unable to experience emotional intimacy. If I empathized with her feelings, it felt intrusive to her and she shut down; if I didn't, she felt rejected and became angry. She felt threatened even if I only reflected something she was feeling, and interpretations were met with denial and hostility. She had a daughter about the same time that my first daughter arrived from India. We talked at length about baby issues, which felt safe for her. How did I feel about getting up in the night to feed my daughter? (Tired but I loved the special time together.) How often did I give her a bottle? (Whenever she was hungry.) What did I feed her? (Goat's milk that I made into formula.) Did I let her just cry? (No!) How was it being a single parent? (She asked because her husband was arguing with her about getting up and feeding her daughter during the night. I told her that no one argues with me when I want to do it, but then there is no one else to get up in the middle of the night, either.)

We also discussed our philosophies of child rearing and she began to talk about her childhood. After a few months of this, she had a dream that signified a turning point in our relationship. In her dream, she was walking in a valley with her hands tied behind her back with rope. She couldn't get free and a voice came over the mountains saying, "Get a goat!" She got the goat, which ate her bonds and she was freed. Sharing my thoughts and feelings about a mutual and less threatening subject had allowed her to trust me and helped her become free.

If anyone thinks they can totally isolate their personal life from their clients, they are mistaken. I remember a client who was a police detective asking me if I'd separated from my husband. How did he know? There weren't two cars in the driveway and there weren't flowers in my office anymore.

A professor in my postgraduate analytic training institute said that he was going to make his office so that it disclosed less of his personal life by having bare white walls, white furniture and no knickknacks. When I jokingly suggested that he ought to wear a white coat, he liked the idea! He also said that he had done a terrible thing when he hugged a client who had just lost his young son. Granted, there are clients who don't want to be touched and there are some for whom it wouldn't be appropriate, but to make no contact a blanket rule is to eliminate humanity from the relationship. If clients can't learn what a relationship is in therapy, where can they learn it?

The client who lived with seven televisions and no real communication was named Mary. One of my training supervisors told me that since we had the same name, "allowing" her to use my first name would create confusion for her as to who I was and who she was. I didn't agree as she was not suffering from the severe pathology where that might be a legitimate concern. What she needed was a relationship, not more distance. As I became convinced of the importance of relationships in the healing process, I practised more humanistically. Just as my therapist needed to teach me how to hug, I taught Mary how to do it.

There are, of course, limits to what I discuss about myself with clients, although I always respect and validate someone's curiosity, even if I don't answer the question. I also may ask the client to look at why they asked and what they think I might answer. I do that less now, though, than I did in my more analytic days.

REGIMEN AND DIET

Dealing with the whole person (the mind and the body) also came to include regimen and diet. The mind and the body are so intricately connected that they can't be dealt with as if they were separate units. What depletes one, depletes the other.

Some time ago I briefly saw a young mother who had been diagnosed with metastasized breast cancer. She wanted to do energy work and I told her that she needed to support the work with nutrition. She was unwilling to change her diet, which was mostly fast food, and chose to not even try. I never saw her again and learned later that she had died. While I felt saddened by her choice, I also recognized that it was hers to make. My experience has been that those who change their diet can make significant changes in their health.

Many years ago, I was seeing a police detective in New York. (The same one who noticed that I didn't have flowers in my office.) He was about 70 pounds overweight, thirsty, urinating frequently and experiencing erectile difficulties. I told him that although he had emotional issues that could be effecting his impotency, diet and health played a major role and these needed to be considered first. I recommended that he see a diabetologist as I suspected diabetes. He was confirmed as being pre-diabetic and I suggested a diet and exercise that brought it under control. He lost the 70 pounds, the erectile difficulties improved, and we continued to work together on the emotional issues.

"YOU CAN'T PUSH A RIVER" (FRITZ PERLS)

One of the hardest lessons for me to learn was that people have a right to choose their own path and go at their own pace. I'm not here to rescue or save anyone. I can offer clients my experience and training, but each person has to decide how far he or she wants to move. This wasn't an easy lesson for me to learn. Being a caretaker by nature, I wanted to help everyone and felt it was my job to drag everyone into health. Only after analyzing and processing my own, unmet childhood needs was I able to let go of that need and allow each person to walk as far as they wanted to go.

During my first year of internship, I was seeing a woman who was unhappily married. One day she asked, "Tell me, should I leave my husband?" She never knew what a gift she gave me with her question. My response was literally a physical one that I felt throughout my entire body. I told her that I could not make that decision for her, that I didn't walk in her shoes, and that I honestly didn't know. I knew what would be best for me, but that didn't mean it would be best for her. I told her that it was hard enough leading my own life, I couldn't lead anyone else's. I could help her explore her feelings and her options, but I couldn't tell her what to do. It was a lesson I have never forgotten.

I ran a couples group that had been together for a long time. One couple felt ready to leave and another couple then decided to go also. While not everyone in the group was ready to leave therapy, the group as an entity was ready to dissolve. One woman got very angry and told me that I ought to keep it together. I told her that I knew exactly how to do that. I would go to the hardware store, buy lengths of heavy chain, lock everyone to their chairs, and give her the keys. She got the idea.

I have also come to trust peoples' sense of self and I respect their inner knowing of themselves. When a person tells me that they are too frightened to go any further, that they could lose control and become destructive, I trust that knowing.

I had a client who told me that if he became really angry, he could hurt me and damage my office. We agreed that since he knew that about himself and since I didn't want to get hurt, he would tell me before he felt he was going to get to that point. During the entire time I treated him, he was always able to monitor his feelings.

Some individuals, though, are not healthy enough to know when they are about to lose that control and, in those situations, I'm very careful.

I saw a young man with agoraphobia who displayed potential homicidal tendencies on a Rorschach test. I was very careful when we dealt with his anger, and when he left treatment, he had expanded his safe area from a few blocks to 25 miles in each direction from his home. He still had many, serious problems, but he had improved his life significantly and was satisfied with the changes.

THE MANY FORMS OF HEALING

Healing can come though many different means. We don't always have to "do something." Sometimes we don't even have to talk.

In my second year internship, I saw a teenager who was fearful and wouldn't talk. One of 11 children, she would come into the session and not say a word. I soon realized that any effort on my part to get her to talk wasn't going to work and I sat silently with her for six sessions. The head of the unit suggested that I read a book during the sessions so that I would have something to do, and while I was not experienced enough to understand how the silence was helping, I knew enough to know that reading a book would be incredibly disrespectful and anti-therapeutic.

This teenager taught me the value of being with clients wherever they are and that, in most cases, their agenda takes precedence. They know what they need often better than I do. After six sessions, the teenager's parents told me that she had changed so much. I did not have a clue as to what had happened, but now I understand that what she needed was the space to just be herself — whatever that was. She knew that far better than I did.

In another example of meeting the client where they are, an 11-year-old girl named Nina came to see me because she was depressed. Her mother told me that Nina was brilliant and beautiful, and that she and her husband had no idea why their daughter was so depressed because everything was "fine" at home.

Nina was intelligent but not brilliant, nice looking but not beautiful, and I knew the mother was having an affair with another client who had referred her. In Nina's sessions, we played cards and drew pictures, and as long as the conversation was about what we were doing, she was talkative. The minute I asked her anything personal, she stopped talking. I took my cue from her and I stopped asking! Weeks and weeks went by this way. I had to fight my need to "do something" and realize that the experience was the something. We were playing crazy eights and I won the game by discarding the first eight cards I'd been dealt.

She was upset that I'd won, and I told her that for me, it wasn't any fun because we didn't get to play for very long, and that was the fun part. Not only was that a new idea for her, but on another day when she won the same way, she was able to say that winning wasn't the point and she wished the game had lasted longer.

Gradually her depression lessened. Why? Certainly not because of any interpretations I'd made — I didn't make any. She taught me that what was healing was being in a safe environment where no one judged her or expected the impossible from her and she could be herself. Sometimes a client just needs to be with you. Even my young clients teach me.

EXPANDING MY SELF

Changes can come through many different types of messengers, and some of them can radically and forever change your life.

When I lived in southern California, I had the opportunity to study with a well-known pet psychic. Working with her not only enabled me to access the parts of myself capable of expanded awareness, it also opened up the metaphysical world to me. Since my connection to her was through my dog, this also showed me that some of my teachers also have four feet and wear fur. Until then I had thought that psychics were a bit loony and that the belief in auras and vibratory rates was crazy. I was clearly traditional in more than my therapy training!

My dog had stopped eating, was having unexplainable seizures, and her condition was becoming critical. My homeopathic vet referred me to one of his clients who was a well-known pet communicator. Although I wasn't sure I believed in it, I was desperate and nothing else was working.

All the pet communicator knew was that my dog, Amita, had a heart problem. I didn't tell her that there was a heart murmur or which valve was involved. I left Amita with her for an hour.

When I returned to pick up my dog an hour later, the pet communicator described which heart valve was defective, the appearance of my house in New York, the neighbourhood games I played with Amita when she was a puppy, the therapy groups that Amita used to be part of, her favourite foods, and other details that she could have only gotten from Amita herself. There was no denying the existence of another kind of communication.

I was so fascinated that I studied with this woman for many years and also trained at the institute where she had been trained. It was my introduction to the world of energy, expanded awareness and spirituality; and it was life changing for me.

As I was exposed to different kinds of techniques in my therapy, I became more eclectic in my practice. I incorporated what I learned in my own treatment and went to a variety of workshops. I began to use the language of Transactional Analysis because it gave clients a way to conceptualize the internalized part of themselves that was still responding to unfinished business from the past. Referring to the "child" in us is a convenient way to symbolize where the feelings came from and what the experiences were that created them. The "critical parent" is shorthand for all the internalized shoulds and oughts we learned, the "adult" is the CEO, and the "nurturing parent" is just that.

My analytic supervisor objected to this, saying that it would confuse the clients and that they couldn't distinguish between the inner child and who they were. I didn't agree with that then and I don't now. In all the years I've practised, I've never had a client who couldn't understand that the language was symbolic. I dealt with my supervisor by just omitting any reference to the Transactional Analysis terms!

MY TOOLS

My techniques now include energy work, psychodrama, psychovisualizations, using childhood photographs, and using different types of extended knowing, to name some. When I work, the left side of my brain is listening to what the client is saying, applying theoretical understanding, and going through a variety of possible interpretations. The right side of my brain is listening intuitively and free floats until something clicks into place and I understand it first emotionally and then intellectually. (It is imperative that the clinician has had good therapy or this part can become severely distorted.) Then I put the two together. This is not exactly what a client of mine thought when he said, "It must be nice for you. You just sit there listening and don't do anything." He should only know!

There are times that I use extended awareness or knowing. Sometimes it is my body that knows, other times I just know that I know something although I do not know where the information comes from. In some way, I have extended my awareness beyond myself and I know something with clarity.

A client of mine who is a homeopath recently told me about a young client of hers who was very overweight and didn't want to go to school. As I was listening, my chest began to feel tight, I was having some difficulty breathing, and I kept seeing scenes of violence. I told this to my client who then shared with me that the young girl had asthma and had witnessed her mother being beaten by her boyfriend. Interestingly, this is what my body had been sensing. It knew before I did.

Another time, a client who happened to be a psychotherapist, was telling me about her client. I told her that her client had been sexually abused as a child. She asked me how I knew, as she hadn't told me about it. I told her that I didn't know how I knew, I just did. It took quite some time and a significant amount of working on my own issues before I could trust that "inner knowing." In order for the therapist to be able to trust that the inner knowing is accurate, he or she must be sure that it is not a reflection of his or her own unresolved, inner chatter. The knowing is only as clear and accurate as they are.

Role-playing and psychodrama are wonderful and creative tools that I have used in many different ways. The various elements of a dream may be role- played for greater understanding. Empty chairs representing people important to the client or different aspects of the self may be used to help the client finish the unfinished business.

Another use of psychodrama involves dealing with an issue. Diane was raised in a deeply religious and conservative family and she carried with her all the shoulds and oughts that she had absorbed as a child. They didn't all fit her adult life and she was struggling to let go of them. I suggested we have a funeral mass for them.

Diane wrote down all the parental shoulds and must nots and put them in a box which was weighted with a brick. At the time, my office was on Long Island near the water, so we went out on a pier, she recited parts of a funeral mass, and we gave the box a burial at sea. Enacting the disposal of the learned, outdated constraints helped her to dispose of them in real life.

PSYCHOVISUALIZATIONS

Psychovisualizations are mentally constructed images or a series of pictures of something that may or may not exist in reality or at that time. In addition to enabling the body to heal itself, psychovisualizations have the potential to reduce fear, anxiety, anger or any feeling that's perceived as overpowering.

A recent client was diagnosed with breast cancer. There were two tumours, each three millimetres in size, and the cancerous cells had spread beyond the margins. She visualized angles in the shape of Pac-men who devoured the tumours and then filled the newly emptied spaces with sunlight.

After doing this twice a day for three weeks, the client had a lumpectomy. The surgeon was surprised to find only one tumour which was less than one millimetre in size. In addition, all the margins were cancer-free, or "clean." The client had used visualizations to trigger her interferon system and to mobilize her own healing powers.

Another recent client was reluctant to try a psychovisualization as he didn't believe that it would work for him. He was very frightened of being alone. It brought back the feelings of emptiness and pain that he had experienced while growing up. The emptiness was visualized as a dark blue balloon that he was able to pop with a pin.

As he loves to garden, he filled the space with a garden full of plants and flowers. He also visualized a bench where he could sit and read. He told me a few days later that, much to his surprise, he still found the garden very comforting and the emptiness was not as terrifying. The psychovisualization had reduced the fear that the little child inside him was feeling, and expanded his adult, capable self.

PHOTOGRAPHS: WINDOWS INTO THE PAST

Photographs can be extremely useful to help clients connect emotionally with parts of themselves or with others about whom they care deeply. Photographs make the idea of the person as a child more concrete and tangible, and the emotions from that time more accessible. I have also used pictures help clients get in touch with long-buried feelings about people who are important to them.

There are a number of exercises I do with photographs. Looking at a picture of oneself as a child helps a person become aware of that child, of what he or she felt and thought. It makes getting in touch with the internal child part of us much easier.

One very powerful exercise is to have the client bring in a picture from childhood and then describe for that child what kind of life has been made for him or her. It helps the client confront who they are and what they want to change.

Another exercise involves having the client tell themselves as a child in the picture what he or she will give that is needed and what will be done to help. This technique can also be used with couples, with each person telling the partner's picture what he or she is willing to do to help that child.

HOMEOPATHY

Homeopathy has had an enormous impact on the way I practise therapy. I was introduced to it by my homeopathic veterinarian when I lived in southern California in the early 1980s. Once again, my dog Amita was the catalyst for my growth.

I became interested in studying homeopathy and have graduated from the Hahnemann Center for Homeopathy and Heilkunst. The remedies and therapy are synergistic and extremely powerful when used together. Not only have the remedies replaced the allopathic drugs that I used to recommend for the clients who needed medication, but they provide help in both bringing up the emotions that need to be processed and in dealing with them once they surface.

Therapy, in turn, processes the feelings that the remedies stir up. A client, who was seeing me for both therapy and homeopathy, came in one afternoon in a panic attack. She felt anxious and had vaginal burning. Knowing the history of her physical symptoms, I knew that the burning was an indication of her anger. I gave her a remedy for anxiety and also one for anger.

While she sipped the remedies, single droplets in a glass of water, we talked about what she was feeling. She was unhappy with her job as an art teacher and felt that her creativity was being stifled. This was reminiscent of her childhood when she wanted to be involved in the arts but was made to be a gymnast instead. After about 15 minutes of therapy work and taking the remedies, her panic was completely gone. I don't think that either the therapy or the remedies would have worked so quickly on their own.

My own experience with remedies has shown me that many of our emotions are held in our bodies on a cellular level, and that therapy is often not enough to release them. I had worked on my own anger and sadness for many years and with many different techniques. While I had been able to release much of it, there was always a layer left. It wasn't until I started taking the remedies and removing my traumas in sequence that I was able to finally release the feelings and work through them. The remedies had made the feelings accessible to the therapy process.

A knowledge of remedies is also important when I work with clients undergoing homeopathic treatment. A client may be feeling sad and lonely which could be coming from something current, something old that is being triggered, or from a remedy which is bringing these feelings up.

A little girl had become fearful, was crying, and had even become reluctant to go outside. I had been treating her sequentially, that is, going back in time over her life and giving her remedies for each successive trauma, be it falling out of bed, starting school, measles or vaccinations.

She had taken remedies for the trauma of physical birth. Her mother had wanted a natural birth and after over 30 hours of labour, she had to go into the hospital where she was given a number of drugs. The infant was vacuumed out with medical machinery.

The child was reacting to the trauma of her own birth as well as to the emotions of fear and anger that her mother had felt. The next set of remedies was for emotional birth and within days of taking them, her fears and crying stopped. I also worked with the mother to help her with her own reactions to the birth. I suggested techniques that would help her daughter, but they wouldn't have been enough without the remedies.

Another client, Mike, was having dreams about the life he led 15 years earlier and couldn't understand why he was dreaming about them. While certainly the dreams were relevant to his therapy, he was taking remedies for events on his timeline that happened 15 years ago. The remedies were bringing up the dream material for healing.

In another case, Monique came into a therapy session saying that she couldn't tolerate having her husband touch her breasts. When I asked her where she was in her sequential treatment, she told me she had taken remedies for something that happened when she was 14. I then asked her what else had been going on at that time. She stopped, thought for a moment, then remembered that was when her breasts had grown quite large. She had been teased about them and tried to keep them hidden, as she was so embarrassed. While she needed to process the eelings, the remedies were the trigger for them.

KARMA AND LESSONS

I have also incorporated my beliefs about karma and life lessons into my work. I no longer think that everything we experience in the here and now reverberates only with experiences from our childhood. These experiences may also be echoes from past lives or they may be the result of karma or life lessons. In the past when clients didn't change, I used to see that as resistance, which is a natural part of therapy and is worked through. While it may be resistance, I now consider the possibility of karma. A client may need to stay on a certain path for karmic reasons, or it may be part of the person's life lesson. When someone has a memory that they don't understand or it doesn't seem to fit into their experiences of the past, I now consider that it could be from another lifetime.

MORE CHANGES

Another change from my traditional training is the way I structure appointments. I was trained that clients who want to reserve a time come in weekly, they are responsible for that time, and not wanting to keep the appointment is resistance (again, not a dirty word). I now have clients who come in when they feel they want to, clients who come in weekly, and some who come in on an as-needed basis. I trust their knowing of themselves and their needs. I'm not sure how this fits into the concept of resistance which is still a component of treatment, but I'm open to seeing what happens.

FURRY, FOUR-FOOTED CO-THERAPISTS

Animals are used in all kinds of helping situations. There are seeing-eye dogs, hearing dogs, rescue dogs, and pets who visit hospitals and nursing homes to name a few. They bring comfort, love and acceptance.

My pets, especially my dogs, have been very important in my therapy work. This is certainly not a traditional technique. I did not consciously set out to use my dog, Amita, in my sessions. She was just so unhappy being upstairs by herself that I brought her into my office, both for individual sessions and for groups. (If clients are allergic or don't want any pets in the room, the pets stay upstairs.)

Amita offered a form of comfort and unconditional love that was safe for clients to accept. Often this was the first opportunity they had to safely experience these feelings.

I was seeing a 35-year-old woman who wore masculine clothing, never had dated, was dyslexic, and lived with her elderly father whom she cared for. She started bringing raisins to Amita, who would run up to her, jumping excitedly for them. One day she forgot them and Amita ran up to her and greeted her just as enthusiastically as she always did. My client started to cry and said, "She likes me anyway." She was able to accept for the first time that she was likable, and I have never doubted that Amita was able to help her experience that far faster than I could have.

My client, Mary, was lying on the couch one day when Amita jumped up, straddled her, and started licking her face. She didn't move but began to cry softly. Finally she said, "No one has ever kissed me like this before."

Amita was often the link between isolation and the first step in trusting me. She also provided me with material to interpret for my clients.

One afternoon Amita was sitting on the couch between a couple who were having an argument. The wife was telling her husband that he didn't pay enough attention to her, and he denied this, saying she didn't notice when he did.

During this exchange, Amita started licking the woman's hand. She didn't mind as they had two dogs at home and were used to it, but she didn't notice it. Amita moved closer to her and kept licking her hand. I didn't say anything for a few minutes then pointed out to her that she was doing with the dog exactly what her husband said she did to him. My words alone wouldn't have had nearly the impact that her experience with Amita had.

Amita also helped in my groups and she was so intuitive that she would just go and quietly sit at the feet of someone who needed to work. It got so that whenever she did that, the person she selected would say, "It must be my turn to work, here's the dog."

Just recently I had my two dogs, one of whom is still a puppy, in a session. They were very restless and unable to settle down, which is unusual for them. My client, Paula, was feeling quite anxious and overwhelmed with childhood, critical messages that she was worthless and incapable. After she put her adult, critical parent, and child each into its own chair and had a conversation between them that culminated with her kicking her critical parent out the door, she felt relaxed and at ease. I looked down and both of my dogs were asleep on the floor. They had mirrored her feelings of anxiety and calm for her.

Over the years, I have had four different dogs in my sessions, and from time to time one of my cats will wonder in.

Elisa was 33 and when she was a young teenager, she had been physically and sexually abused by her brothers, one of whom she found electrocuted in the bathtub when she was only 13. Trusting was difficult for her, and she was working on the feelings she had about her parents' failure to protect her from the abuse. She was feeling cold and distant and too frightened to deal with the issues. Shashonna, one of my cats, made a rare appearance in my office, walked over to Elisa, and spent the rest of Elisa's session draped around the back of her neck like a scarf. Elisa felt warmed and protected and became more able to take in what I, a mere human, had to offer.

One of my clients, who has dealt with a tremendous amount of trauma in her life, was talking about her fear of selling her house which she and her ill husband could no longer afford to keep. Making changes was very difficult for her, as it is for many people. Canna, one of my rescued cats who was so frightened that she lived in my basement for eight years before she felt comfortable enough to come upstairs and who rarely appears around strangers, meowed until I let her in my office. She sat quietly in front of my client, as if to lend her support from one who knows about the fear of change and the possibility of conquering that fear. (Canna now sleeps next to me on my bed.) When my client was ready to talk about another issue, Canna left. My cats seem to know exactly when they're needed and stay only for the time that the need exists. After that, they just slip out of the room.

MY WORK, MY LIFE

I also learned to incorporate the circumstances of my life into my work.

When I was living in New York I injured my back and had to lie almost flat for about a month. I set up a lounge chair in my living room and saw clients there.

Everything that happens is grist for the therapy mill and lying on my back during sessions certainly gave my clients a lot to process. All of my clients needed to deal with what it meant to them to have me lying almost prone in their sessions as well as meeting in my home instead of my office. This was especially significant for one client whose mother had always been sick and unable to care for her. Not only was she able to get in touch with how she felt when her mother was so ill, but she was also able to experience that not everyone who is injured is as incapable of caring for her as her mother was.

TANGLED SPAGHETTI OR WHAT EXACTLY IS THERAPY?

Almost every client who is new to therapy has asked me "What exactly is therapy?" It's an important and valid question. The only problem is that I've never found a really adequate explanation. I can explain it technically, but to convey the emotionality of it is impossible. Long ago a client likened therapy to untangling a plate of wet spaghetti, and that is a good analogy.

Some people resist psychotherapy and choose it only as a last resort, when their emotional pain has become too great to bear. Unfortunately we come from a cultural background that teaches us to pull ourselves up by our bootstraps, have a stiff upper lip, and go back to work. Dealing with emotions is often seen as a weakness and an indulgence. Why is it we would never consider trying to fix a broken bone ourselves but we expect ourselves to be able to heal a broken heart? We think that we should have the skill to deal with our emotions ourselves and that anything that has to do with feelings is just common sense. Psychology is a body of knowledge and psychotherapists have extensive training. They are as expert at helping you heal a broken heart as medical doctors are in fixing those broken bones.

Therapy involves the re-education of the knowing, adult part of us, as it observes and participates in the processing of old child-like feelings, beliefs and misconceptions. Therapy is not just an intellectual process. Knowing and understanding are important, but not enough. You cannot build a house without a blueprint, and you can't live in it, either. It is the emotional processing that is the true work of therapy, and I believe that requires openness, creativity, trust in the client, and a willingness to share of oneself.

Therapy also requires that the therapist has been well analyzed. You cannot take anyone to a place that is unknown or frightening to you. I am always alarmed and amazed when I meet therapists who have never had therapy. How can people possibly understand the process without having experienced it themselves?

If a client is stuck, it's often because the therapist is stuck. I had a client who was so terrified of his anger that even asking him to tell me about a sword that appeared in his dream caused him great fear. Nothing I did seemed to help him open this door into himself. I presented his case at a conference (sound familiar?) and role-played him. At one point, when I was being him, I moved my hands in a particular fashion and literally stopped mid-sentence. My hand gesture reminded me of my sister, and after I worked through the similarities I was experiencing between my client and my sister, I was able to help him become "unstuck."

Therapy is a mixture of head and heart, of knowing and feeling. It requires the willingness of the client to take some long-untravelled roads and the willingness of the therapist to have gone there first.

WILL I RECOGNIZE MYSELF WHEN I'M DONE WITH THERAPY?

How much change will there be? Will I still be myself? People naturally wonder what therapy will do for them and to them and frequently ask "Will therapy change who I am?" Let me answer that with a story.

The man who knew that if he became very angry he was capable of hurting me worked hard in therapy and made significant changes. He got married, was able to control his anger, developed more self-esteem and self-confidence, and was promoted in his job. He came in for his last session, sat down, and told me that he was really angry with me. I asked him why and he said, "I thought I'd come out of therapy a new person. I'm still the same person, I just handle everything differently." Then he realized what he'd said and laughed.

After therapy, you are still essentially you. The adult is stronger, the critical parent is much quieter, and the child is less fearful. On a good day when the sun is shining, the old scars are not even noticed. On a bad day, you feel them but they don't incapacitate you any more.

AND HOW LONG WILL IT TAKE?

The other big question clients ask is, "How long will I be coming to therapy? How long will it take?" I saw a couple many years ago who got up and walked out during the first session when they learned it would take more than one appointment.

I tell clients it all depends on how thorough they want the changes to be and how fast they go. I remind them that there are 8,760 hours in a year and it will take some time to work through the 20, 30, 40 or more years they have been alive. It has been said that children are like modeling clay, but adults have already turned into concrete and it can sometimes take a jackhammer to loosen them. I wish it went faster, not only for them but for my own growth as well. It takes time, though. As a client of mine said recently, "I'm under construction."

Therapy is not intended to last forever. Its goal is to help people work through enough problematic feelings so that they can function better and use the tools learned in therapy to continue to grow on their own.

Therapy is a wondrous journey and I am privileged and honoured to be able to accompany my clients. I am in awe of the resiliency of the human spirit, the drive for health and the courage my clients continue to show me each day.

It has been a privilege to share these stories with you. I wish you well on the path of your own healing as your mind, heart and soul open to all the wonders that are possible for you.

Acknowledgements

This chapter is dedicated to my daughters, Mara and Maya, who have stretched me and expanded my understanding of myself, my clients who have taught me so much, my therapist and mentor, Larry Vogel (1924-2003) who gave of himself so that I could become more of myself, and all my pets who have been my co-therapists and teachers.

Last of all, thank you to Serena Williamson who encouraged and inspired me to write this chapter.

– Mary Rothschild

Chapter Five

Your Body of Knowledge
Back to You

By James Emmett, BSc, DAc, MMSc, DC

About James Emmett

Dr. James Emmett, a 1994 graduate of the Canadian Memorial Chiropractic College in Toronto, was moved by his patients' unexpected emotional responses to traditional chiropractic care. His quest for deeper answers brought him to Dr. Paul Lacroix, his mentor and friend, who showed him what it was to love chiropractic and encouraged his true role as a primary contact practitioner.

Dr. Emmett's understanding of healing deepened further on meeting Rudi Verspoor. Impressed by the success of homeopathy for himself and others, Dr. Emmett studied Heilkunst for a year to learn more about it.

Sequential homeopathy fuelled a desire for knowledge that took Dr. Emmett to new areas of healing. He studied craniosacral therapy for three years and subsequently integrated those specialized techniques into his regular chiropractic practice.

During one craniosacral course Dr. Emmett met Jocelyne Couture, a practitioner who works with energy medicine. Jocelyne has demonstrated the effectiveness of this type of work again and again. This further broadened his knowledge base.

Dr. Emmett met Rania McKinley, a medical intuitive, while attending a seminar in Philadelphia. Medical doctors send patients to her for a second opinion or for a confirmation of their diagnosis. Meeting Ms. McKinley was another opportunity for Dr. Emmett to discover what is available outside of our traditional way of thinking in applying treatments.

To understand the application and benefits of acupuncture Dr. Emmett studied with Dr. Sir Mehran Hakimennegad. He also travelled overseas to study acupuncture with Dr. Sir Professor Anton Jayasuria at the hospital in Colombo Sri Lanka.

Dr. Emmett considers these experiences as the tip of the iceberg with respect to what we need to know about our health and our bodies. Dr. Emmett has found that learning one skill that can help people opens ten more doors for learning opportunities.

Dr. James Emmett can be reached at:
Centrum Chiropractic and Acupuncture Clinic in Ottawa, Ontario.
613-830-4080
DrEmmett@bellnet.ca.

YOUR BODY OF KNOWLEDGE
Back to You

O ur bodies are wonderful testaments to our lives, embracing both what we inherited from our parents and ancestors, and the way we live now. Stretch marks, stress lines on the face, back trouble, irritable bowel along with hundreds of other conditions not only tell others about our life and lifestyle, but also remind us what we should or shouldn't continue to do to our mind, body, soul and spirit. Thus, your body has the knowledge of experience from physical, mental and emotional events.*

As a practitioner it is my job to help the patient unlock the truths from their body to allow them to begin their healing journey.

BEGINNINGS

My mom was a nurse, my dad a metallurgist. My sister is a nurse, counselling mom and dad on their medications and diet practices. My brother has a degree in biology, has worked as an orderly, and recently retired from the pharmaceutical

---

* As you can well appreciate, the names have been changed or abbreviated for any patient referred to in this chapter.

industry after 17 years, as he once described himself in jest, as a "drug pusher." At the time of writing my brother has been accepted into his first year of Nursing at Queen's at the tender age of 41.

Uncle H was a nurse, then a psychometrist. Both Aunt B and Aunt H were nurses. Uncle B is a psychiatrist. My cousins D and JR are medical doctors. Another cousin is medical researcher and her husband is a chief anesthesiologist.

With this type of family history it is no wonder that when growing up, my siblings and I never had scrapes and bruises, we suffered abrasions and contusions. We never cleaned a wound we had to abrade it. Going to the bathroom meant doing our ablutions. This all seemed normal to me until people started commenting on the unique quality of that behaviour. To this day my mom can describe in clear detail antiseptic and sterilization procedures to help prevent post-operative infection.

I have had hospital visits for many broken bones and my fair share of needles, surgeries, concussions, physio appointments, mercury fillings and antibiotics.

After high school I enrolled in Carleton's Engineering Science program and spent two years there. It was an unfulfilling experience, devoid of personal warmth and "natural" interactions. Next was Kinanthropology — human movement studies — at the University of Ottawa. Courses included anatomy, physiology, sports psychology, exercise prescription design and biomechanics among others. Upon graduating with a BSc, I took a year off working for a sales company learning a lot about people, their money and the fact that I would never do that type of work again.

Returning to academics, I was accepted at Queens for my MSc in exercise rehabilitation. Studies were medically based and encompassed hospital work and maximal treadmill testing of elite and weekend warrior athletes.

Inundated with three decades of personal and academic science and medical exposure, how is it possible that I finally came to be where I am today?

THE CHIROPRACTIC JOURNEY

My chiropractic experience started with a neck injury during a high school football practice. I had a helmet-to-helmet hit with our middle linebacker. The only difference in our head positions was that Mark's hit me with his head centered between his shoulders, and mine was tilted towards the right. Upon contact I immediately felt a "pop" and lack of movement in my neck. Over the next several hours and into the next morning it continued to worsen such that I was unable to turn my head in any direction, or look up or down. With no other option apparent to me, I went to see my MD. After his examination, he suggested I see "this guy" just down the street. No mention of the word chiropractic was made. Just "this guy."

So I arrived at the chiropractor's office with no clue to what I was supposed to do and say. Taking a history and conducting a thorough exam he broke the news to me. I had a subluxation at the fifth and sixth segments of my neck. A sub-what?!! What do you do, cast it? "This guy" told me that a simple adjustment was all that was needed.

Following the first adjustment of my life I experienced 75 percent greater movement in my neck. Several more adjustments over the next few weeks and I returned to 100 percent. Continuing with care on a preventative basis would have been the best thing to do, but I had to wait many more years to discover the benefits of that.

Some years later during my second year at Ottawa University I began looking to the future and found myself unsure about what to do after graduation. It was my friend JZ, in dating a chiropractic student studying at Canadian Memorial Chiropractic College (CMCC) in Toronto, who re-directed my curiosity to chiropractic.

I needed to find out if chiropractic was for me. In my last year of Kin-anthropology I was able to do two electives. For the first elective I volunteered with a physiotherapist/athletic therapist, C.W., who taught me a lot about rehabilitation of injuries and sports medicine. To me it seemed too mechanical and routinized, and although I was always learning, it was simply not dynamic enough.

In the second elective, I completed an internship with Dr. M., a chiropractor who had graduated just a few years earlier. I became his patient and it became apparent that regular adjustments were improving my overall health and mobility. Dr. M. gave me assignments for reading, allowed me to develop x-rays (at that time it was hand-dipping x-ray processing) and to observe patients being adjusted. It was amazing to see someone come in with significant headache symptoms, and see that same person leave with a smile, headache relieved. I would consistently see his patients' symptoms improving.

It didn't take long to realize this was the dynamic career I was looking for, and now I knew it was what I really wanted to do.

In 1990, I began my first-rate education at the CMCC. Courses were taught by chiropractors, PhDs, medical doctors plus graduate students and they were interesting and varied. As part of our graduation requirements we had to be involved for one year as a junior intern and then a full year as a graduating intern.

Following academic and clinical-competency final exams for school, there were Canadian board exams. These exams were tough — nine exams in five days. After that there were provincial oral, practical, x-ray and written assessments. I graduated in 1994 and returned to Ottawa that same year.

After graduating from CMCC I felt I was aware of the holistic experience that the patients needed. But I was still in the mini-medical mindset. This created a philosophical dilemma for me until I had a chance to talk with Dr. Paul.

I met Dr. Paul 18 months after graduation. He shared with me his philosophy of chiropractic, his love of the profession, and his love of helping people return to health through adjustments. For me, this marked the major step toward the "bigger picture" using chiropractic care as the guide.

In school we were taught about the innate wisdom of the body, but it wasn't until I met someone who lived and breathed chiropractic that it all came together. Now I understood why the model of health that I was given while growing up, and which had never felt quite right, could no longer be true for me.

My truth is "new." My truth is about the body, the beautiful self-regulating, self-healing body that has no spare parts for removal and which has no deficiency of aspirin. Everyone knows it, but few ascribe to the fact that health does not come in a bottle.

My truth is about life and its experiences — either good, better or best. My truth is about that sweet core of the soul that we are born with and how it changes with each and every mental, chemical, emotional or physical event, be it big or small.

My truth is about the happenings of your past and your present and how to improve your future health for the sake of yourself, your family and children, and future generations.

Chiropractic can help with all of these things.

There are many ways to deliver chiropractic care. In fact, there are more than two dozen techniques with which to adjust the joints of the body.

There are many chiropractic practitioners doing a wonderful job and changing the world "one spine at a time." The way I approach chiropractic is neither right nor wrong, better or worse than anyone else's approach. It is just my way.

From my first day of professional chiropractic practice almost ten years ago, it has never ceased to amaze me the lessons I am taught, each day, from every single patient. Some lessons are very clear right from the beginning while others are still unfolding, even years later.

WHAT IS CHIROPRACTIC?

The purpose of the nervous system and the spine is to control/regulate and receive feedback from every organ, muscle, tissue and cell of the body. Any interference along a nerve will interfere with the function and control of the respective organ, tissue or cell. Subsequently, since every part of your body is related neuro-humerally — i.e., the relationship of the nervous system to the hormones — to every other part of your body, any interference with the nerve will adversely affect your physical, mental and social well-being.

Chiropractors call this interference along a nerve a subluxation of the spine or other joint of the body. The subluxation complex involves two vertebrae and the disc in between, or two opposing joint surfaces. It is this subluxation which affects our health. Chiropractors remove subluxations from the body through the adjustment to help restore the body to health. After an adjustment you can become clearer in thought, more mobile, healthier, and generally more interactive overall.

This subluxation complex consists of five sections. The lack of proper movement of the joint, *kinesiopathology*, can result in lack of motion or hypo-mobility, compensation of the body, and possibly excessive joint movement or hyper-mobility in surrounding segments. Included with this can be *myopathology*, or muscle changes where the contractions may become spasms to protect the affected joint and the muscle may become fibrotic. The nerve irritation or pressure, *neuropathophysiology*, creates sensory changes, changes in blood flow or muscle spasms in the former, or weakness or sensory loss in the latter. *Histopathology* indicates that local swelling is taking place with biochemical changes occurring as the local joint environment is altered leading to degeneration. The *pathology* that results can be seen in organ or body system dysfunction.

Through the adjustment, the innate wisdom inside each one of us is allowed to fully express itself, providing us the opportunity to make our state of health more complete. It is the adjustment that chiropractors use to eliminate subluxations from the body. Chiropractors adjust the spine to remove subluxations, thus restoring spinal function, and taking the individual towards optimal health.

Having started chiropractic adjustments and care for their designated spinal complaints, many patients comment on so-called "unmentioned" health improvements. On the initial chiropractic history and examination, numerous patients thought it unnecessary to mention such symptoms as heart burn, asthma, allergies, constipation or diarrhea. After a short time they discover to their delight that as their spinal health improves so do their other conditions.

... get knowledge of the spine, for this is the requisite for many diseases.

– Hippocrates, the Father of Medicine

CHIROPRACTIC – UP TO DATE

B.J. Palmer the "Developer of Chiropractic" wrote:
Chiropractic is a science of the cause of things natural; not a science of symptoms; not a science to chemically analyze the constituents of the human body (normal or abnormal). But it is the science of how to analyze certain conditions quickly back to the cause, and we only utilize conditions in so far as they exist as a guidepost or mile-post on the road, telling us purely which way we must go.[1]

---

1 Rondberg, Terry, D.C., *Chiropractic First, The Fastest-Growing Healthcare Choice ... Before Drugs or Surgery*, Chiropractic Journal Publishing, 1998.

The cause that B.J. refers to is the effect of improper spinal movement, the subluxation that causes pressure on a nerve. Subluxations can be located anywhere along the spine, also in the shoulders and ribs or in any joint of the body. Pressure on a nerve causes an increase or decrease in organ, tissue or cell function wherever that nerve supplies innervation. Thus, if the organs are affected your optimal health status will be disrupted.

In 1895, Daniel David (D.D.) Palmer, B.J.'s father and the founder of chiropractic, adjusted the spine of a deaf man only to have that man's hearing restored. The Canadian-born D.D. (Port Perry, Ontario 1845) spent several months after this first adjustment correcting spinal misalignments and improving his patients' health, calling them "hand treatments" before coming up with a term for what he was doing. Eventually he and his pastor derived the name we use today, *Chiropractic*, from the Greek words *Chiro* meaning hand, and *practic* meaning treatment or operation. The major tenet of chiropractic is that an Innate Intelligence or Universal Intelligence exists within our bodies, giving it, the body, properties and actions. It is this Innate Intelligence, found within all matter, which allows the body to function. The Innate maintains the existence of all matter.

Most people believe that chiropractic is relatively new. However, the practice of adjusting spines goes back perhaps to 17,500 BC, and is definitely recorded in China (2700 BC), ancient Greece, and in the ancient American Indian civilization. B.J. Palmer took the work of his father and developed the present-day art, science and philosophy of the chiropractic profession.

Since its inception in 1895, chiropractic has had its challenges. A number of chiropractors, including D.D. Palmer, had been jailed for practising medicine without a licence.

In New Zealand the chiropractic profession was considered an "unscientific cult," which in 1979 led to a Commission of Inquiry into Chiropractic. That commission found that *"Chiropractors should, in the public interest, be accepted as partners in the general health-care system. No other health professional is as well qualified by his general training to carry out a diagnosis for spinal mechanical dysfunction or to perform spinal manual therapy."*

More recently in 1990, the American Medical Association was found guilty in a District Court decision of having created a conspiracy amongst its members and other health-care organizations to systematically destroy the credibility of the chiropractic profession.

Even today the Chiropractic profession faces ongoing challenges. Sensationalist stories in print and on television create fear and doubt about chiropractic within the public eye.

When the medical profession publishes a report, or someone denigrates chiropractic in the media, the overwhelming sentiment of the patients at my clinic is "here they go again." Chiropractic patients see the bias quite clearly.

Despite the obstacles that the chiropractic profession has faced over the years, chiropractic is still the number one chosen drug-free "alternative" health-care choice.

In Chiropractic First [2] Dr. Terry Rondberg details numerous research studies from all over the world that demonstrated either the safety and/or the efficacy of chiropractic care. How much evidence is enough before governments recognize the benefits of chiropractic care and make it fully covered under provincial insurance?

THE INITIATION TO THE BODY OF KNOWLEDGE

The new patient examination of Sandra was complete. All the orthopedic, neurological and chiropractic procedures indicated that this was not a complicated case. Posture was fair to poor in the neck and mid-back. Muscle palpation or tissue feel, showed over-tight neck muscles, not uncommon for someone with a computer-related occupation. Palpation of the joints of the spine — called facet joints — showed disruption of movement, and the fifth and sixth cervical spine segments were particularly tender to the touch. The range of motion of her neck was limited by pain, most notably in rightward rotation.

X-ray findings demonstrated a reversed cervical spine curvature (no longer c-shaped in direction). No evidence of disc disease, no evidence of breakage or

2   ibid.

collapse of any bones, no tumours or calcifications. The diagnosis was a facet irritation or biomechanical lesion or subluxation — all terms of the same meaning — to the fifth and sixth vertebrae of the neck. This situation was explained to Sandra and she understood the condition and long-term consequences to her neck and overall health if this problem was left untreated. The enviable safety record of chiropractic was noted as she signed the consent form to begin care. Sandra was ready for her first adjustment.

What happened next was something that my years of training could not have prepared me for. After a specific, light adjustment to her neck, Sandra broke into tears. The tears did not come from pain, but as she described it, came from someplace completely different.

THE PART OF THE WHOLE PICTURE

We never know how far-reaching something we may think, say, or do today will affect the lives of millions of people tomorrow.

– B.J. Palmer

For centuries we have been fed medical dogma about our health through seminars, books, radio, television and commercials, magazines and now the Internet. Top of the list is the notion that the body can be separated in distinct sections and thus treated accordingly: stomach pills, liver pills, sex pills, joint pills...the list goes on and on. There are heart doctors, ear, nose and throat doctors, cancer doctors, gastroenterologists, orthopaedic doctors and foot doctors.

I once had an acupuncture patient with severe prostatitis who reported receiving medication to eliminate only the constant burning he was experiencing, whether urinating or not. The rationale was that if the burning was gone then the prostatitis must be getting better. The burning decreased but he was developing stomach pain, headaches and other physical changes as side effects.

The ever-increasing reliance on equipment and technology to "find the problem" will allow greater advances into understanding the phenomenally minute details of the body. However, this will also lead most people farther from the truth of the big picture – the ability and vital importance of seeing the whole person as a union of mind, body and spirit.

This is where the chiropractor plays a key role. The doctor of chiropractic comes in to bridge the understanding for the patient that everything is indeed connected from above down and inside out. The chiropractor or "body doctor" tries to see the whole picture. There are many examples to illustrate this, but using one from my intern clinical experience will suffice.

A female patient arrived at the walk-in clinic complaining of headaches that had persisted for many years. General examination revealed some postural changes witnessed as a lateral deviation of the spine or scoliotic curvature, causing or the result of one foot which being moderately pronated or simply the loss of arch height. She was fitted with orthotics (custom designed shoe inserts) and over the course of the next several weeks, with neck and full spine adjustments, the headaches disappeared.

Most people want to know how the foot was connected to the headaches. The flattening of the left foot caused several things: a drop in the pelvic crest height at the belt level; tightening of the supporting low back muscles; compensation in the mid-back area between the shoulder blades causing a drop of the right shoulder; imbalance and tension of the muscles up to the neck, and subluxation of the upper cervical spine creating the headaches.

The orthotics corrected the foot biomechanics, lifting the arch of the foot and thus allowing all segments of the spine to be approximately level. Once level, the dysfunctions or subluxations in the spine needed to be corrected. That was done through the adjustments.

This patient got the results she was looking for, improved her health and quality of life with no medication, and was free from side effects. She was not subjected to invasive procedures, just the whole body perspective and chiropractic care.

THE FIRST VISIT

The overall assessment of the patient begins the moment he or she enters the clinic. First-time patients complete an intake questionnaire. Occasionally I am near enough to the front desk to quickly observe the patient filling out this form. This brief viewing is sufficient to give me an impression of not only the level of pain, but also the comfort level with the clinic and environment, the look of fear in some cases, the severity of the problem, or even the level of stress present. This is evident in and expressed by facial expression, position of the head, neck and shoulders, the way the arms hang at their sides, how they write on the page, or hold a briefcase, how they position their knees, feet or even what they have done with their shoes once they are off. I have made connections with certain types of behaviours and conditions simply by close observation.

The look of the patient and the feeling that is experienced from them as I enter the adjusting room is very important. The impression given as they stand to shake hands, including how their body reacts to light touch and what they talk about (or not talk about) during their treatment time — these are all clues about their personal bigger picture.

The cause of a patient's pain is often locked deep within their body. I find that during clinical interaction, hints of it will come up in general conversation either before, during or after the adjustment. They don't necessarily have to say anything. The cause, or factors contributing to their current physical status, will often be written all over the body usually with posture, facial expression and eye clarity. Usually the picture presented on the outside is a result of the "stuff" going on at a much deeper level inside.

Self-knowledge is not bestowed on us; it must be gained through experience and participation.

– Frank Rivers[3]

3   Rivers, Frank, *The Way of the Owl: Succeeding with Integrity in a Conflicted World*, Harper San Francisco, 1996.

INTERESTING INSIDES

All people have within their inner natural resources a powerful ally, their higher self, which sometimes tries to teach them things about themselves by manifesting particular types of illness or dysfunction.

– Richard Gerber, MD[4]

The body is truly amazing. From the way we walk to the way we chew food, each and every function is related to our overall health. When disrupted, functional mechanics of the spine and limbs can cause not only disturbances in surrounding tissues but also dysfunction and altered health conditions elsewhere in the body.

Every system of the body is connected to every other system. Every cell is related to every other cell. Every day our nervous system and brain are bombarded subconsciously and consciously with millions upon millions of signals about our external and internal environment. The body takes the necessary measures to receive the input, analyze it, interpret it, then sends out the new signals for the body to adapt. Innate Intelligence makes this adaptation possible, and the result is the way that we express our life, our very existence.

In chiropractic, this life force is called the Innate Intelligence, the life within the body, the inner wisdom. This inner wisdom is that which allows cuts to heal, bones to mend and the heart to beat faster when someone says "I love you."

Despite the best efforts of the scientific community, there has yet to be a laboratory experiment using the food that someone may take in over breakfast, lunch and dinner to create all the hormones, blood cells, sweat or bones that are the necessary requirements of daily living and bodily functioning for that individual. The Innate does all of this.

The Innate performs body functions, day in day out, regardless of our attempts to intellectualize and scrutinize. The body lets us know when we need to intervene or lessen our interference. At the basic level, when we are hungry or thirsty, messages are sent to eat or drink.

---

4   Gerber, Richard, MD, *Vibrational Medicine: New Choices For Healing Ourselves*, Bear And Company, Santa Fe, 1996.

All of our life experiences — mental, physical or emotional in nature — shape the way we input information, with good or bad experiences skewing our analysis and interpretation, and then we react accordingly. The physical reaction or symptoms is the one most widely recognized.

Chiropractors have begun this understanding since the first adjustment D.D. Palmer performed at Davenport, Iowa in 1895. It became a little clearer in the early 1900s when B.J. discovered the neurocalorimeter. That was a device to assess spinal function and corresponding nerves as they relate to internal organs. Thus the relationship between the spine and the entire body was becoming more apparent. Acupuncturists, some chiropractors, massage therapists, homeopaths and energy workers recognize the whole body connection. Many medical doctors are also starting to see the bigger picture.

Studies that have examined the immune system have found that following a regime of chiropractic care, there is an increase in levels of T and B lymphocytes (carried in the blood along with NK cells) antibodies, phagocytic activity, CD4 counts and plasma beta-endorphins.

These big words basically say that the cells that fight body-invading viruses, bacteria, toxins and even organic waste, get a boost with regular chiropractic care. Many patients also report a decreased susceptibility to colds and flu.

The adjustment itself is a powerful tool to help release not only physical blockages, but also any resistance due to many stored-up emotions including anger, happiness, sadness or fear.

Intelligence is present everywhere in our bodies…our own inner intelligence is far superior to any we can try to substitute from the outside.

– Deepak Chopra, MD[5]

EMOTIONS

Only through emotions can you encounter the force field of your own soul.

– Gary Zukav[6]

5   Chopra, Deepak MD, *Quantum Healing: Exploring the Frontiers of Mind/Body Medicine*, Bantam, New York, 1989.

6   Zukav, Gary, *Thoughts from the Seat of the Soul: Meditations for Souls in Process*, Fireside, New York, 1994.

Early in my chiropractic career I was doing a locum for a colleague when one of his patients came in complaining of severe low back pain. There were no falls, accidents or injuries to have created such severe pain. All orthopedic and neurological tests performed on this patient were negative. Reasonable range of motion of the low back was demonstrated. Other than extreme tenderness over the bones of the low back, everything appeared to be within normal limits.

As we discussed the findings of the examination, somehow the conversation veered towards his home life. Something in the conversation prompted the comment from me, "I think you have to resolve the tension and problems within your relationship with your wife in order for the low back pain to improve." Neither right nor wrong to say it, yet there it was, with no take backs. I have no idea why I decided to say it, but it came straight from the heart, with no filters. He didn't challenge me on that statement, just sat quietly and looked at me rather tensely, becoming very pale and then softly indicating he wanted now only to be adjusted. He continued with chiropractic care at the clinic but I never saw him again.

Sometimes the direct truth is too powerful. Now if that same type of patient comes to the clinic and a similar truthful thought comes up, I wait on it, and attenuate it accordingly. I have since discovered that the patient must discover what "their real truth" is for themselves. By asking the client questions, and helping to answer theirs, they find their way to self-discovery of their truth.

For many years Jane had received chiropractic care initially for low back pain. The pain would resolve nicely and then she would go about her way, only interested in pain relief, not interested in maintenance or supportive care of any type. Over the time I had the opportunity to work with her, it was obvious that she was incredibly stressed both at work and home. This showed up as a tight rigid face, stiffness in body movement, diminished shine in her eyes, and terseness in her voice.

One day she suddenly came out with, "Do you think this has anything to do with stress?" I agreed that it did. Then I recounted to her the different things she had mentioned in passing over the last several years about events going on in her life. When you speak from the heart, people listen.

"Well, my neck is getting really sore recently. Could it be from my husband?" We both laughed out loud. I laughed again inside, not at her, but her pain in the neck connection with her husband. "I feel I am not listening to my body. If I don't listen soon this is just going to get worse. My god, what am I going to do, if I don't take care of myself now?"

We discussed the idea of adjustments improving not only her immune system but also the improvements she may notice in her stress levels with supportive chiropractic care. Supportive meaning that chiropractic care is received when there are no symptoms. Many patients find these regular adjustments effective in maintaining their mobility, dealing with life stress more effectively, and for a generalized sense of well-being.

This was one of those "aha" moments that led Jane into a sequence of emotional revelations and many questions concerning her health. She began acupuncture and is considering starting homeopathy, all for the purpose of improving her overall state of well-being.

Chiropractic allows the opportunity for people to be relieved from pain, sets the rigid body in motion and helps the poor outlook on life start to become rosy again. With a healthier person, their internal energy flows more naturally and more positively. As these people become more positive, they smile more and become healthier. Through chiropractic care, their interactions with people are filled with more love and compassion.

FAST FOOD "HEALTH" CARE

We do much damage by not being patient with our own evolution, which by design and necessity luxuriates in an abundance of time and plot twists.

– Greg Levoy[7]

Drive-through burger places, speed dating, drive-through banking, and drive-through flu shots. How much can I get and how quickly can you get it to me? Society is all about immediacy and immediate gratification with long-term consequences being of no concern.

---

7   Levoy, Greg, *Callings: Finding and Following an Authentic Life.* Three Rivers Press, New York, 1997.

"Patience, be patient. The improvements will come." I say when interacting with the patient who isn't. But they don't have time for that. Most everyone wants it yesterday, whatever "it" may be.

Many people view their health in the same "deal with it quickly" mindset. I don't blame them. Inundated with so much from TV, movies, music videos, radio, etc., you can't escape the pressure to follow along, particularly if you have never been given or seen any other health options. Many times other healing options are dismissed as "quackery" by friends, family, or someone in the medical profession, regardless of their knowledge about the subject.

People need to get rid of that rash, and quickly. Little do they know that putting on cortisone cream suppresses the cause of the rash, and the disease which caused the rash will be expressed somewhere else in the body as a lung congestion or some type of diagnosed virus or "flu." But at least they'll look good. But what is it at a deeper level that is "getting under their skin?"

Headaches are gone fast with over the counter medications, but without a deeper understanding of how the person's environment, home life, chosen occupation or lifestyle is affecting them. Surgery for the tonsils or adenoids is done with little thought to the immune system regulation changes that will take place. For a long time the appendix was thought to be "just an outgrowth" of the large intestine. Now there may appear to be immune function to it, but also suggestions of a predisposition in males to prostate problems as a result of an appendectomy.

Antibiotics for childhood ear infections are given without looking at the child's spinal health. Sometimes it is the lack of resonance in the relationship between the parents which can cause the problem. This puts a lot of pressure emotionally on a child and ear infections will pop up. In these cases, the parents along with the child should have some sort of intervention. This is where it is important for the practitioner to observe, listen and feel for the environment around the child.

In a health lecture given by chiropractor Dr. Steve Marini of the International Chiropractic Paediatric Association, he discovered some interesting feedback from parents in the American Medical Association design to get the chicken pox vaccine to market. What he found was the main driving force for the implementation of the vaccine was to delay the onset of the attack of the chicken pox. The delay was necessary for the child to be old enough, in university or out of the house so that the child could be self-sufficient. The parent wanted a way to avoid the sickness out of convenience sake so that they would not have to take time off work to look after a sick child.

Although a lot of these conditions and their medical treatments are described as commonplace this does not mean that they are natural or effective. The end goal with medical treatments/interventions of course is to improve "health" as they see it. But what is missing is the thought of why, from a deeper level did this particular disease show up in the first place? Understandably a quick high spike in body temperature is dangerous, but what is the purpose of fever? What does that action of suppressing a fever do to the child's immune system in the long run? What has been suppressed in that child that will be expressed later somewhere else in the body?

Little thought has been given to the long-term detrimental effects of such decisions on the child's health. The medical association has lost sight of the beneficial effects that most childhood illnesses and fevers have on priming the immune system so that it becomes stronger, naturally.

Where has the accountability gone for one's health, or our children's health?

Most everyone wants someone else to be responsible for every aspect of their well-being. Some people will make a token effort towards health, such as joining a health club or starting the "newest" diet. But once the hard part begins, the novelty wears off and they are back to their old habits again. Almost everyone wants immediate health gratification, even if the problem has existed for many months or even years in some cases.

Numerous patients suffering from carpal tunnel syndrome come to the clinic for chiropractic or acupuncture relief of their problem. A number of them wanted to avoid having another wrist surgery, but this time on their "good" wrist. Upon further questioning a large portion of these patients reported that the surgery was only mildly successful the first time. Carpal tunnel syndrome can be a result of nerve compression in the wrist, elbow, shoulder or a subluxation of the cervical spine creating irritation of the nerves that run down into the hand.

But from a soul-spiritual level, what is the body of knowledge trying to tell the person suffering from carpal-tunnel? What are you holding on tight to?

What anger is causing you to clench your fists?

These factors must be observed by the chiropractor subtly, and without judgement. The care must be directed not only to the physical manifestations, but also carefully and quietly towards the treating the deeper issues. Helping the patient to find out what they need to do to complement the chiropractic care being received is of great importance.

Manon came to the clinic for acupuncture complaining of bilateral carpal tunnel syndrome. This woman was very stressed, depressed and anxious all at the same time. She was so out of touch with her own body that the only symptom she recognized was wrist pain. Acupuncture care was directed to diminishing her stress, calming her down and boosting up her immune system. We never worked on the wrists. After two weeks her carpal tunnel was completely gone and only flared up, worsened to 10 percent of the original pain, when work got very hectic.

Chiropractic, acupuncture, nutritional intervention, homeopathy and massage therapy are all techniques that we use at our clinic to help carpal tunnel and many other problems.

We all have evolved to where we are today based on our life experiences. The direction of our evolution has been dependent on what we do with our experiences and from what we learn from them. If you do not like the direction of your current health status, what are you doing, not doing, or not facing in your life or work that is helping to create the problem? The more challenging the experience, the more we can learn. The universe never gives us more than what we can handle. Life is not a drive-through. Your health is not a drive-through.

Each of us tends to think we see things as they are, that we are objective.
But this is not the case. We see the world, not as it is, but as we are —
or as we are conditioned to see it.

– Stephen R. Covey[8]

8   Covey, Stephen, *Seven Habits of Highly Effective People*, Simon & Schuster, New York, 1990.

YOUR BODY IS SHOUTING

To take in a new idea you must destroy the old, let go of old opinions, to observe and conceive new thoughts. To learn is but to change your opinion.

– B.J.Palmer

What did your body say to you throughout your day? What does that mean to you? What does it say about the way your life is currently going? Is there a consistent theme to your illness? A timing pattern with respect to your illness(es)?

The chiropractor has to listen to the accounts of the patient's history of injury, while at the same time trying to listen in between the words as to what else the patient's body is whispering, speaking or shouting that the patient knows about, but has yet to hear or realize. Listening is a state of being. Sometimes it is important to be alone and quiet to help understand your state of being. Looking deeply at the patient helps me to listen more attentively.

If our bodies are overloaded from stress, there will be a point the body shouts out "No more stress" and shuts down. This has happened to a number of patients. In particular, a patient Gina, experienced this very event. She is not in a resonant relationship and it is stressing her to her wit's end. She has never spoken directly of the relationship, but it is obvious in her body language, her eyes, hair and general demeanour, plus the feel of her spine and rib cage. Gina moves her underweight body rigidly and cautiously, trying to control every move. Her eyes are sad and bloodshot. The red lines throughout the whites of her eyes indicate severe mental overload. Her autonomic nervous system and her body's endocrine system have been working too hard. Her body is stressed.

Both the autonomic nervous system and to a lesser extent, the endocrine system, balance the internal environment of the body. The nervous system has been directly correlated with the function of the endocrine system, which in part determines this homeostasis. Briefly, the autonomic system is concerned with rapid changes, while the endocrines' secretion of hormones causes mainly slower and more precise control of the body functioning.

Although Gina is always well presented, her hair looks tired and lifeless. All x-ray findings show adequate joint and discal spacing, but her body is rigid and stiff to the touch. Due to the stress overload that her body was demonstrating it was important for her to switch from the traditional hands-on chiropractic care to the hand-held instrument called the activator. For Gina, this was significantly more comfortable and effective.

Through the chiropractic adjustments, the nervous system supply to organs, tissues and cells is optimized. Subsequently the endocrine and autonomic systems can be influenced by these same chiropractic adjustments to help normalize the bodily systems.

Gina had been regular with her adjustments over the last number of years, but the decline in her overall health took place over the course of approximately six months. Her adjustments had also becoming farther and farther apart. Although she denied any problems, she did complain of stomach pain, bad taste in her mouth and squeezing pressure around her chest.

Gina hadn't been in for several months, and showed up one day at the clinic. Whatever was happening in her life had finally culminated into a seizure, from which she spent several weeks in hospital. There was no medical diagnosis for this event but she was given anti-convulsants as a precaution and released from the hospital.

Gina is a little more together now. She comes in for regular adjustments and is seeing a sequential homeopathic practitioner. She is still in the relationship and she is a little more assertive, expressing to her partner what she requires. She has gained some weight, her nutrition appears better as her hair has more shine to it. Gina has slowly started an exercise program and has begun her own home business.

Sometimes it takes a health crisis such as the one Gina experienced for people to take action and move in a healthier direction; for example, the man who starts an exercise program because of a heart attack or the woman who loses weight because of her severely high blood pressure. Why do we wait until we are lying in a hospital bed for someone else to tell us to be healthy?

Our bodies first whisper a symptom about an upcoming problem. Then the body talks. If we still have not shown the respect the symptom expects, the body shouts.

Then look out! If action is taken upon the body's shouted request for attention, the shouting is attenuated or muted altogether, usually followed by low-grade murmuring. It is the one without wisdom who returns to the old health patterns, ignoring the shouts, and that is when the echo hits.

How do you listen to your body?

A symptom only ever corrects imbalances: the overactive are forced to rest, the restless prevented from moving, the sociable cut off from all contact. The symptom forces into the open the pole that we have been failing to live out.

– Thorwald Dethlefsen [9]

THE HOMEOPATHIC JOURNEY: I'LL SEND MY WIFE

Two years after beginning chiropractic practice, I decided that I wanted to supplement what I was doing for my personal health. A chiropractic patient, Linda, spoke glowingly of a sequential homeopath she had consulted. She was talking about Rudi Verspooor and the Center for Heilkunst.

Heilkunst treats the deep underlying causes of disease and imbalance through bio-energetic homeopathic medicine in combination with diet, exercise and energy therapies. These remedies are given in a specific sequence dealing with the significant mental, emotional and physical shocks and traumas of a person's lifetime. Treatment begins with the most recent event, moving back in time to the individual's birth process and perhaps into the treatment of what the sequential homeopaths call the miasms or genetic predisposition.

Linda was in the clinic for a follow-up adjustment several weeks later and she was talking again of this homeopath, Rudi. She was very convincing this time. I was curious. But I still had that bad experience in the back of mind. So I did whatever a good husband would do, talked it over with my wife Kris, got her opinion and then I sent her to see Rudi.

---

9   Dethlefsen, Thorwald, *The Healing Power of Illness: The meaning of Symptoms and How to Interpret Them*, Element Books Ltd., Boston, 1990.

Kris came back with glowing reports and told me: "You've got to go see him. He is very interesting. He looks at you when you talk and he listens." She is a very good judge of character. I went to see Rudi and am so glad I did. He has provided me with a whole new perspective on health.

Since starting homeopathy the Heilkunst way, its path to healing has led me to study acupuncture, muscle energy techniques and craniosacral therapy. It has allowed me to grow and expand in my knowledge base and as an individual. Through it I have met some wonderful and healthy people and practitioners. Without Heilkunst I would never have had the opportunity to create with the very interesting co-authors of this book.

Heilkunst has allowed me to discover a health perspective not only for myself but also created a perspective shift as I look at my patients. I look at patients a lot differently than when I first began my practice. I look at myself a lot differently as a practitioner than when I first started. As an interesting note, I have observed that people who have undergone sequential homeopathy therapy have different sounds to their adjustments than those who have not had homeopathic care. Their adjustments have a crisper, cleaner sound to them. Their eyes are clearer and there is less tension to their bodies and spine. The adjustments are easier to do.

I have been so impressed by what I have seen with homeopathy that I attended classes and studied this practice for over a year. My wife completed her postgraduate work in homeopathy, a process that took over three years.

SPARKLING EYES

Many beautiful words have been written about the eyes. Numerous people have called them "mirrors of our soul." Eyes not only provide us with the perception of our surroundings but also show to others what is within us, from the outside looking in.

Chiropractors have a quick view of overall health and are given an idea of the state of mind of the patient simply by making eye contact. Connecting with each patient, including children, with a handshake and eye contact does wonders for their overall experience and for the perception of the care that they are to receive.

I love the sparkle and depth of the eyes of someone who is fully alive — fully alive with health, love, joy and wonder. Many children display this love, wonder, excitement and yearning for knowledge that makes their eyes sparkle, dance and sing. What is it about our living that lessens or strengthens the sparkle? How does that happen?

When I first met Janet and Bill in 1996, they were a funny spirited couple who came to the clinic to receive adjustments not only for their aches and pains but also to remain mobile and so that would "not appear their age." What made them even more special was that they were in their late 80s. Chronic health problems had taken a toll on Bill. His eyes were not clear and his posture was poor. Janet had few health complaints, but she had the sparkling eyes of a child.

With their age as a factor, Bill having a history of cancer and Janet being a very petite woman, we agreed to adjust them with the hand-held device, the activator. The activator allowed us safe and effective adjustments to their spine and peripheral joints. In combination with stretches, muscle work and the activator, their aches and pains diminished but Bill's eyes never showed any improvement in clarity. Janet's continued to shine.

Although at that time Bill had been cleared of any cancer, I felt somehow that it was returning. They continued to be patients at the clinic on a maintenance/supportive monthly basis. When they would go to Florida for their six-month migration, they saw a chiropractor there.

Two years after our first meeting and as a result of cancer, Bill passed on. As could be expected, Janet was crushed, but she wasn't defeated. Her eyes dulled a little. But her spirit came back to be as strong as ever.

Since the death of Bill, Janet has suffered a number of injuries, for which she has come to chiropractic for help. She has strained the rotator cuff of her shoulder, fractured ribs on her right side, fractured ribs on her left side, and fractured her sacrum all in separate falls. For these injuries Janet has been treated with chiropractic care, acupuncture, craniosacral and muscle energy techniques. She heals remarkably quickly.

Janet is now 94 years of age, as feisty and fun loving as when I first met her. She still comes in for her monthly chiropractic adjustments and care. She is the "honorary" grandmother to my daughter Avery, which made Janet's still sparkling eyes even brighter.

MR. T & ME

Early in my chiropractic career I was in a multi-chiropractic office during regular hours when a patient of another practitioner came in with obvious distress. I read the chart for his previous history, type of chiropractic care he receives and looked at the x-ray reports of the most recent films taken. He was a new patient to me, so I had to become acquainted with him, his spine and his condition. A complete chiropractic examination was conducted.

Mr. T. was diagnosed with an uncomplicated cervical spine facet joint irritation/subluxation. There were also subluxations in his mid and lower back.

Mr. T. was a 75-year-old German Second World War veteran, a large man, with a very bad limp, a result of a bomb blast during the war, other shrapnel wounds to every part of his body, and he was missing several fingers on each hand, but he held a warm, generous smile. Mr. T. had received chiropractic care for many years, but over the last several months his treating chiropractor had difficulty adjusting his neck due to stiffness, resistance or for other reasons yet unknown. He made a point of telling me this, so that, I assumed, I wouldn't be too upset if the adjustment didn't work for him on that particular day.

He lay down on the chiropractic table and I palpated the tissues of his neck. There were subluxations, one vertebrae up high on the left side of the neck, and the other lower down on the right.

As part of our graduating requirements for school we required a lot of clinical experience as chiropractic interns. This experience was garnered in a controlled academic environment, where the patients were relatively calm and who usually went quietly on their way. That was not what happened on this day.

Mr. T. was set into the adjustment position and … click. His neck was adjusted. Immediately Mr. T. sat bolt upright, grabbed his neck and yelled in his thick German accent "Oh my god, oh my god!!!" To say the least, I was startled. Before I could say anything he continued with, "it hurts but it feels so good!!" Then he jumped off the table and started running around the room in his limping gait, around me, around the table, around me, around the table again and again and again exclaiming loudly "it hurts but it feels so good!" I just sat there speechless, watching him go around and around in his underwear.

After what seemed like an hour, but I am sure it was only a minute or two, he began to calm down enough to lie down on the table again. We discussed briefly what had happened and he confessed that this was the first time in a long time that his neck had been adjusted and he was caught a little off guard. It hadn't really hurt at all.

Now it was time to check the neck again, after the adjustment, with palpation. There was much better movement and reduced subluxation at the segment adjusted. Only one more vertebrae to adjust…click.

"Oh my god, oh my god" up and running in circles again went Mr. T., but this time in the other direction around me, around the table, around me, around the table again and again. In another couple of minutes he was calm again. His thoracic spine or mid-back and lumbar spine or low back, were then adjusted without incident. Mr. T. was so happy about the success of his neck adjustments that he referred his wife, son and daughter to the clinic. They all enjoyed a measure of success with chiropractic.

A BROKEN SPINE

… a kind of super intelligence exists in each of us, infinitely smarter and possessed of technical know-how far beyond our present understanding.

– Lewis Thomas MD[10]

During my first year of practice, Mary, a teenager, came to the clinic for a new patient consultation. She walked into the clinic treatment room with a full frontal upper torso cast and low back cast, in separate pieces held tight to her body by

---

10 Rondberg, ibid.

elastic bandages. Mary was a tremendously gifted volleyball player who had suffered a stress fracture to one of the lower vertebrae of her spine.

Mary had been warned by a hospital specializing in children that not using the cast properly and taking it off too early would be extremely detrimental to her spinal well-being. She was also told that her volleyball days were over. Mary was depressed, frightened and apprehensive about "going against doctor's orders." After all, she did have a broken spine.

A full chiropractic examination, utilizing chiropractic, orthopaedic, neurological testing plus a standing x-ray examination was completed. The diagnosis concluded that she did in fact have a fracture, called a spondylolysthesis at the fifth vertebrae in her lumbar spine, but this fracture was held in its usual place by the supporting spinal ligaments. It was considered stable. This was all good news for Mary's situation.

With Mary's case, however, research at that time indicated that casting for the fracture that Mary had suffered was counterproductive. The first thing she needed to do was to eliminate the use of the cast. Her postural supporting muscles had become weakened. The muscles of her trunk, which included her stomach, sides and back, needed to be re-educated to function properly again. The vertebrae of her spine needed to be adjusted and corrected, as there were multiple subluxations of her spine.

Chiropractic care began with only the Activator technique, trigger point therapy, and soft tissue therapy to her trunk stabilizing muscles and she was given mild core strengthening exercises. Over the next three months Mary gradually progressed from the Activator method through to drop table work and then to full spine, hands on adjusting.

Mary was able to begin training for volleyball again and went on to star in high school volleyball. She also starred in university volleyball and was honoured to play with the Canadian Team for one set of an exhibition game. Pretty good outcome for someone who was told five years earlier that her volleyball days were over!

Imagine a boulder rolling down a hill. If you try to stop it with direct force or with dogged resistance, you will be defeated. But if you run up along side it and give it a nudge in a new direction, you will remain safe.

– Frank Rivers

CHILDREN KNOW

When I approach a child, he inspires in me two sentiments: tenderness for what he is, and respect for what he may become.

– Louis Pasteur

Newborn infants' lives, from the adult perspective, for the most part seem quite easy. Or are they? Initially they live in the warm cozy environment of the uterus that eventually becomes too cramped. All too soon it is time to move out, but in order to accomplish this, the child must move down a tunnel, twisting along the way to avoid getting the shoulders stuck. The tunnel is tight and the cranial bones of the head are squeezed into a partial cone shape.

Each of the bones of the skull has an independent movement and rhythm. This rhythm of movement is present in everyone and is independent of heart rate and respiration rates. This cranial bone separation of the birth process which is important for the movement/massaging of the cerebral spinal fluid down the length of the neural canal. If the cranial bones do not return to the original position after birth, health symptoms may show up.

Then the presentation of the head occurs. Following this event the usual mode of extraction of the infant out of the birth canal takes place. This is usually where the first subluxation of the spine happens.

Other techniques of removal including vacuum extraction, forceps, and caesarean births can create their own set of problems; problems caused by faulty relationship of the cranial bones, possibly resulting in visual problems, respiratory or digestive difficulties to name a few.

A poor repositioning of the cranial bones may give the infant's head an irregular shape. Craniosacral therapy has worked wonders to help return cranial rhythm to normal, restore the balanced look to the skull, and eliminate health problems associated with deficiencies of cranial bone movement.

I attended a cranial seminar where one of the participants brought in her child towards the end of the seminar day. The baby, less than one year old, had a head that was noticeably flattened on one side. The seminar leader, Nina C., a massage therapist and craniosacral specialist, asked permission to work on the child, noted the history and began to work delicately on the head of the child. After approximately 20 minutes of work, Nina had to do no more therapy on the child. Her head had returned to a "normal" relatively symmetrical shape.

I have told this story many times, and received mixed reactions. Some people do not believe the story. Their minds are already made up after being told by "authorities" that that is just the way the head ends up, nothing can be done, and the child will have to live with it. Others want to hear more and then take the appropriate steps of action for their own child, and share the story with other friends or family.

Once the infant is out into the world, all new stresses and strains begin to happen to the body. From neck positioning while breastfeeding, to sleeping on Mom or Dad's shoulder to the way they are picked up from the crib, all have effects on the spine of a child. Infants can't tell if they are crooked or if their spine is affected. Several times different parents have brought their infants in to the clinic, saying that there has been no bowel movement for several days. A check of the spine indicated subluxations at the upper lumbar segments of the spine. After specific light activator adjustments, the infant either had a bowel movement immediately while in the clinic or within the next several hours when at home. Follow-up appointments are always recommended to ensure continued spinal alignment.

Chiropractors are criticized routinely for their desire to adjust everyone from infants to seniors, criticized for what the dental, medical, or optometry authorities espouse as prevention. Does the nervous system not supply the teeth with sensation? Isn't it the optic nerve that allows us to see? The nervous system was in place before the eyes developed in the womb or the teeth popped into our mouths.

The tremendous importance of the spine and its development is well known. If a child has scoliosis – a lateral deviation of the spine, sometimes it is picked up early and the "monitoring" of it begins. Being asymptomatic as most scoliotic curves are, it may go unnoticed for years. It is the role of the chiropractor to assess the look and function of a child's spine. Why is an adult's fully formed spine more important to adjust than a spine that is just beginning to grow?

Children are adjusted all the time at the clinic. They intuitively know what is good for their health. Many children want to be adjusted before their parents and siblings and often compete for who will be adjusted first.

How refreshing it is to hear a parent say that their four-year-old daughter had a tummy ache, didn't want any medicine but wanted to go to the chiropractor for help. A number of parents even bring their children in to the clinic when they start to become too hyperactive and won't settle down.

Chiropractic adjustments help calm or remove nerve irritation (subluxation) at the spinal level. Once the nerve is less irritated, the organ, tissue or cell at the end of that nerve also begins to settle down and so too may the child.

Children need chiropractic care for a variety of reasons. All the falling, tumbling and rolling they do can lead to subluxations. They need chiropractic care to help them grow straighter. Adjustments of the spine can correct subluxations affecting nerves that control the organs or tissues leading to asthma, allergies or tonsillitis, tummy aches, bed wetting or urinary incontinence. Adjustments may be given to correct subluxations created from the stress of the birth process. The application of chiropractic is so easy and complex at the same time.

Yvonne was a new patient at the clinic. On one particular visit she started talking about Stewart, her 18-month-old son who was having a problem with his ears. He was now on his fourth round of antibiotics for ear infections. This is a common thing to hear at the clinic. We scheduled an appointment for Stewart for later that same day.

In Stewart's case, his examination revealed a subluxation or dysfunction of the first and second vertebrae of his neck. This type of problem can create a variety of health issues such as congestion in the head, lack of proper drainage from the ears, lung irritation or stomach and digestive problems. It was suggested to Yvonne that quick and significant action must take place to eliminate this problem. Yvonne agreed since the medical doctor, who had looked in Stewart's ears just that morning, said the eardrums were very red and swollen. Due to the severity of the eardrum swelling Stewart was to see the MD again in five days for a follow-up.

Stewart was adjusted twice a day for five days. Yvonne started him on specific vitamins, a modified diet to decrease his sugars and hard to digest food, and he was given acidophilus daily, a product to help restore the intestinal bacteria destroyed by the antibiotics.

Yvonne recounted the story of the next MD appointment, which will remain with her for a very long time. After the five-day interval, facing them in the examining room once more, the MD picked up her otoscope and looked in Stewart's ears. She pulled the scope out, shook her head and looked into his ears once more. The ears were healthy looking again, no more swelling, no more redness. "All clear." The MD stated. "Yes they are, thanks to chiropractic!!" Yvonne replied, gathering Stewart up and quickly leaving the office.

How many people go through this cycle of antibiotics, time and again only to have tubes placed in the child's ears? They are never given any other options. Research clearly shows, in medical journals such as the *British Medical Journal* and the *Journal of the American Medical Association,* plus others, that antibiotics including amoxicillin are ineffective for the treatment of ear infections. In 2000, the Agency for Healthcare Research and Quality found that 24 hours following the diagnosis of an ear infection, the pain and fever were gone in two-thirds of the children, without the use of antibiotics. Within seven days, still without antibiotics, over 80 percent recovered.

As is starting to happen, a groundswell movement is occurring of people who are demanding a change in the direction that our so-called "health-care" system is going. Intuitively, people the world over are beginning to sense and understand that what their MDs are telling them with respect to their treatment or health status is confusing and ineffective. They don't quite know what it is wrong, but they know that something is not as it should be. But they do know what they want, health care that is natural.

There was that law of life, so well and so just, which demanded that one must grow or pay more for remaining the same.

– Norman Mailer

AND THEN …SILENCE

My daughter Avery was just over one day old when she had her first adjustment. The lay person may say "What, are you crazy! Kids, especially infants, don't need chiropractic. It's too dangerous to do that!" Chiropractors reading this chapter might ask me, "What took you so long?" but excitement of being a new dad, holding Avery in my arms and looking into her eyes, plus fatigue and all the other factors, didn't have me in that "adjusting" frame of mind.

It wasn't until the very early hours of Avery's first full day "out" that her relentless crying was concerning both my wife Kris and me. Kris held her and walked with her. Avery breast-fed. No change, crying continued. We gave her homeopathic remedies, her cry softened a bit but she continued.

Avery kept crying, and crying quite loudly for a one-day-old. "What can I do? What can I do?" I kept asking myself. Then it hit me, "I'm a chiropractor, check her spine and adjust her if necessary."

I assessed Avery's little spine as carefully and precisely as possible. There were subluxations in her spine at the base of her skull. They were the result of birth trauma. This type of trauma is similar to that which most babies experience in a natural birth, with a short or long labour.

Luckily enough and with no preplanning in mind, my activator was on my nightstand right next to the bed. I reached over and grabbed it, set the activator on a setting suitable for infants and Avery was adjusted at C2 on the right side of her neck, and C1 on the left.

Instantly, and I mean quick as a blink, Avery stopped crying and fell asleep. It was as if someone had turned off the crying button. The silence was now very loud. The irritation was off the nerves of her spine, the joints were back in place and the pain was gone. She could now relax and fall asleep.

At the time of this writing Avery is 17 months old. Very articulate for her age, she calls the activator Daddy's *click clack*. Avery is checked for subluxations every couple of weeks, and is adjusted along her whole spine as the assessment dictates.

When she sees the activator in my hand, she comes right over smiling and she sits on my knee patiently waiting for the *click clack* to happen.

Beautiful. Healthy. Natural.

> *A child's world is fresh and new and beautiful, full of wonder and excitement.*

> – Caroline Norton

JAMES – IN "HYPER SPACE"

> *You have to be able to determine what the axis of condition is for the patient,*
> *then the appropriate steps must be taken to remove that axis.*

> – Rudi Verspoor

James was 10 years old, easily distracted at school, couldn't or wouldn't do his homework, started missing classes and then started shoplifting. The teachers wanted him on Ritalin. He needed to be calmed down, so he would be easier to teach. They said he was ADHD.

Six months prior to these events, James had been a "normal" nine-year-old boy who was getting along with everyone, paying attention in class and doing his homework. The parents were defiant in the knowledge that their son was not ADHD. They brought James in to the clinic for an assessment.

Dr. Brian Abelson,[11] DC, RNC has researched Ritalin and has discovered some interesting facts. Ritalin and cocaine are classified as controlled Category 2 pharmaceuticals. Cocaine has biochemical reactions and properties similar to Ritalin.[12] Ritalin is manufactured and consumed in the United States five times more than the rest of the world combined. Ritalin decreases the flow of blood to the brain

---

11 Dr. Abelson can be contacted at www.drabelson.com.

12 "Methylphenidate," DEA Press Release, October 20,1995.

by 20 to 30 percent, and there is a concomitant decrease in cognitive functioning.[13] Ritalin causes symptoms similar to Parkinson's Syndrome. The diagnostic criteria are highly subjective and varied, requiring a direct observational period of at least six months. Are they really confident that this approach is the best answer?

James' history revealed no falls or traumas to his body over the last number of months. His assessment revealed postural changes of his head, on his shoulders, anterior head carriage, rounded shoulders and a subluxation of the first and second vertebrae of the neck.

When the brain begins to form the nervous system at the entry level into the spinal opening, part of the brain stem also enters the upper reaches of the spinal canal. If you consider the first two vertebrae as the gatekeepers to the entire system, having their function disrupted for any number of reasons will create a variety of symptoms. The symptoms include but are not limited to: headaches; congestion in the head; stomach trouble; intestines feeling "off"; heart palpitations; jaw irritation; facial irritations; and in some cases, over-activity.

Having a subluxation at that level of the first and second vertebrae is somewhat similar to the reaction of your body when you hear nails scratched on a chalkboard. Your body at a deep level is being irritated to do something but consciously you don't know what. Subsequently you are restless, and your body just wants to keep active because those vertebrae are irritating nerves that go to the entire body. That is exactly what James was experiencing.

All James had was a subluxation. This subluxation created a powerful irritating effect on his whole body. The irritation on his nervous system was so great that he couldn't concentrate or sit still as he was receiving "let's move" messages.

James was adjusted three times during the first and second week. By the start of the third week he was sitting in class appropriately, doing his homework without incident at night, and had apologized and begun to do volunteer work for the man from whom he stole.

A 10-year-old boy, no drugs, no long-term side effects on his body and back to himself again with the love of his family and chiropractic adjustments.

---

13   Breggin, Peter R., MD, Director of the International Center for the Study of Psychiatry and Psychology and associate faculty at the Johns Hopkins University Department of Counseling.

We make a living by what we get, we make a life by what we give"

– Sir Winston Churchill

STEPHEN'S STORY

If you don't take a look, you will continue to be a victim of your own myopia.

– Frank Rivers
The Way of the Owl

Stephen was only 10 years old when he was struck by a car while riding his bicycle. He was knocked unconscious and received many bumps and bruises, but was saved by his helmet, which was dented severely. The headaches, migraines and visual disturbances started soon after.

Since the age of 10 he has been on daily migraine medication to control the serotonin levels in his brain, a cerebral vasoconstrictor, Amytryptyline, as a precautionary drug and daily doses of two Advil and two extra strength Tylenol. None of this has helped. Along with the trauma of his accident, these attempts to control Stephen's internal biological and physiological milieu most likely have created a toxic load on his system, with the drugs overloading his liver cleansing ability and creating problems within his spine (a subluxation).

The nervous system travels from the brain down the spinal canal and out to all the surrounding tissues, cells and organs, then feeds back from the organs to the spine, nervous system and then to the brain for subconscious monitoring. The feedback from the organ to the spine, the viscerosomatic loop, if disrupted, has been found to alter the ability of the vertebrae to move properly, creating a subluxation at the respective spinal level.

For Stephen, his was not a problem that would be solved quickly and might even show up as larger health problems in the future.

CT scan and MRI tests were all normal. His EEG (brain wave assessment) indicated abnormalities in function, a result of the contusion to his brain from the accident. On doctors' advice, Stephen had to give up swimming and basketball.

Now it was five years later and these headaches and migraines continued to be so incapacitating that Stephen was unable to complete homework or even go to school on some days. Wendy, his mother, reported that prior to the accident Stephen was only sick once, with a couple of ear infections as a baby that cleared up with antibiotics. The medical doctors have given up on him. Thankfully, an MD had suggested acupuncture and this is how he ended up at my clinic.

Stephen and Wendy came to see me with significant reservations. A self-described skeptic of anything non-medical, she wasn't about to try anything her medical doctor had not suggested. She only ever wanted Stephen to have acupuncture, so that is what she'd discuss.

Stephen demonstrated some interesting physical signs. His head was asymmetrical, one eye was lower than the other, and he had a recessed chin and an overbite. I told Stephen that I was also concerned for his liver, given all the medication he had been taking for such a long time. The liver has an effect on the eyes as well.

Considering Wendy's defensive facial expression and body language, with caution and respect I began to discuss some of Stephen's physical "deformities" with them. Wendy wasn't buying any of it. She challenged everything I said.

"If what you are saying is true," Wendy began with a scowl and folded arms, "why didn't the MD or neurologist notice these things?" Good question.

I continued. The helmet that he had been wearing at the time of the accident saved his life. The trauma of his head hitting the ground caused a disruption of the cranial bones. This often results in a distorted look to the skull and various effects on the jaw. This disruption affected the dural membrane that attaches to the inside of the skull and surrounds the nervous system all the way down, attaching to the sacrum which is identified as the triangular bone located between your buttock cheeks. From inadequate movement of the cranial bones, tension can be given to the dural membrane and headaches, visual changes and many other conditions can result.

This same type of disruption can be seen in infants with forceps deliveries or vacuum extractions. Although infants cannot verbalize a problem, they do give physical signs such as ineffective suckling, crying relentlessly, high-pitched crying or listlessness. Most of these situations can be related back to ineffective cranial bone movement.

With gentle, delicate pressure on the bones of the skull or other parts of the body, using specific hand and finger placement, alterations in cranial bone, or sacral bone rhythm can be detected. This rhythm, independent of heart rate and respiration, is present in every body and is the result of the ebb and flow of cerebral spinal fluid around the central nervous system. The technique is called craniosacral therapy (CST) and was developed by an American osteopathic physician about 80 years ago.

I gave Wendy and Stephen an introductory book on craniosacral therapy.[14] The entire interaction was subject to a lot of skepticism, so I did not know whether I would see them again.

Two weeks later Wendy called for craniosacral work. "I don't know if it will work, but we'll give it a try." Wendy told Jose, my front desk assistant.

Two sessions over two weeks resulted in better sleep and a reduction in medication and headaches for Stephen. After five more sessions the visual disturbances had started to abate. Stress of schoolwork and life continue to cause the occasional aggravation but in less than two months, Stephen states that he is 75 percent better than he was before starting. Wendy has since started acupuncture for a shoulder and neck problem.

CST is becoming more widely known and is now a remarkably effective treatment option for pain and rehabilitation. It has proven to be beneficial for the treatment of birth and other traumas, learning disabilities, ADD, ADHD, developmental delays, autism, headaches, tinnitus, jaw syndromes, stress disorders and many other pain and neurological conditions.

Our Innate Wisdom, our inner doctor, can alter the physiology and thus heal the body. By removing skepticism around whatever issue is blocking them, the patient is then able to internalize their information. Once internalized, the truth then becomes easier to find.

---

14 Upledger, John E. DO, OMM, *Your Inner Physician and You*, North Atlantic Books, Berkeley, 1991.

CIRCLE OF LIFE

On a Monday in May of 2002, my daughter Avery was born. I saw her head pop out, I heard her first babbling sounds, I guided the rest of her body out of the birth canal, cut the umbilical cord and held this new life in my arms while my wife Kris was being attended to by the mid-wife.

Holding Avery close, I spoke softly to her as she stared intently and deeply into my eyes. Even though she was only minutes old, I would ask her questions and when I paused for her answer, she would blink, as if in understanding. What a wonderful moment in time to cherish. I felt her in my heart. I felt her in my soul.

We had lots of help at home, so I returned to the clinic on the Wednesday of the same week Avery was born, to continue adjusting patients. Little did I know of the day to come!

The clinic day was busy. Everyone wanted to know all the details of the birth. From chiropractic to acupuncture and craniosacral sessions, there was a full day planned.

One of the clients, Mr. Des, had been a patient of the clinic for several years, but since assuming ownership of the clinic, I had only made his acquaintance over the previous several weeks. Mr. Des was experiencing low back pain, for which he was receiving acupuncture.

On this particular day, he was more quiet than usual. When I asked him if he was all right he confirmed that he was. After setting the needles, something seemed off with him so I asked my front desk assistant Jose to check in on him every ten minutes or so. Over the half-hour Mr. Des was in the clinic, Jose had checked on him several times.

At the end of the half-hour session the needles were removed, and we arranged a follow-up for his low back in two days. I then went about my regular routine with other patients.

Ten minutes later, Jose knocked on my treatment room door to tell me that Mr. Des was not feeling very well. I immediately went out to see him in the waiting room. His skin colour, body posture and eyes told me something was not right at all.

We had a brief discussion and started toward a treatment room where he could lie down where a further assessment could be conducted in private.

Just as we stepped into the treatment room, he looked at me and said "I'm going to die" and collapsed. I caught him before he was half way down, held him tightly and lowered him to the floor. With help from another patient, we performed CPR immediately. He died right there. I had heard his last words and his last body sounds. At 83 years of age, Mr. Des diedof a massive heart attack right in my arms.

Some people get the chance to bring life into the world and witness the miracle of birth. Few people have someone die in their arms. Fewer still have both happen in the same week. That week and these experiences I will remember forever. Interestingly enough, two weeks prior to this incident I had changed the quote on the quote board hanging in the clinic. It read:

The source to the soul is through your heart.

– Source unknown

LAST RESORT

"Almost two thirds of Canadian adults suffered from back pain in 2002....

The impact of back pain on the daily lives of sufferers ranged from time off work and difficulty concentrating, to restricted family and physical activities and depression."[15]

Back pain costs Canada 8 billion dollars per year, so it is incredible to believe that the utilization of chiropractic is so low, and the amount of funding for chiropractic care is so small. The efficacy has been amply demonstrated and thankfully every year 4.5 million Canadians use chiropractic services amongst Canada's 5000 chiropractors or the costs could be much higher.

The patients come to the clinic and tell me they have tried everything to relieve their low back pain. That everything, however, does not usually include chiropractic for some reason. The muscle relaxants, painkillers and anti-inflammatories are temporary measures. Most everyone is concerned about how the rest of their body will be affected by continued use of these medications. They

---

15 *Life in Canada a Pain in the Back*, Health Canada National Survey, June 25, 2003.

just didn't know what else to do.

Many patients have received massages whose healing effects, although pleasant, did not seem to last more than a day or two. Others have said the same for home exercise and physiotherapy.

In 1993, Dr. Pran Manga, an economist at the University of Ottawa conducted a meta-analysis of previous research studies that looked at effectiveness and cost effectiveness of medication, bed rest, physiotherapy and chiropractic on low back pain. The results were surprising to everyone else but the chiropractic profession. Chiropractic was found to be the most effective and most cost-effective strategy.

People are hesitant to try chiropractic for a number of reasons, but the real reason is often fear of the unknown.

Some people fear they will become dependent on chiropractic and will "have to go all the time." My response has consistently been: "Once you sense your body moving more freely, your pain goes away, and you start becoming healthy, you become more body aware. You will want to get an adjustment when you start to feel ill or run down, because you will feel the difference in your recovery ability. You know you will need an adjustment before, after or during stressful times, because you know that your head will be clearer, your muscles less tense and the stress will fall off you faster. Your sense of body awareness will return."

Is anyone really stress-free? Why wouldn't you want to be as mobile, flexible and as healthy as you can be for as long as you can be?

Those who are meant to hear will understand.

Those who are not meant to understand will not hear.

– Confucius

WHY DOES MY BACK HURT, DOC?

What a loaded question!

Throughout the previous sections I have tried to show that there are many reasons — mental, emotional and physical — which can cause pain in the body.

When interacting with patients it is important to be aware of these many causes and deal with them specifically. There is not one schedule of care into which every patient must fit. Nor should there be one that binds the patient into some form of contract of care. Each patient is individual and should receive the care that is tailored to their mental, emotional and physical needs.

I consider the spine from the base of the skull down to the bottom of the buttocks all part of the "back" and from there, break it down into sections. I also try to incorporate the ideas and principles associated with a number of different disciplines including homeopathy, acupuncture, craniosacral and chiropractic into the care that the patient receives.

Those who have studied Heilkunst sequential homeopathy have found there to be an emotional map of the body. Simply put, pain in any of the four major segments of our spines – cervical, thoracic, lumbar and sacral – is the physical expression of underlying mental or emotional happenings.

The cervical spine or neck, consisting of seven vertebrae, is the area where we hold our anger. Each of these seven bones and the discs in between hold different emotions ranging from resentment to feeling non-deserving.

The deeper spiritual basis of neck pain according to Narayan Singh is "Anticipated aggravation."[16] Someone with neck pain is experiencing irritation, displeasure and pique about a real or fantasized transaction which is expected to result in some form of attack on their situation, system or self." Basically, someone or something is being perceived as a pain in the neck.

The emotional map relating to the thoracic spine, twelve segments or twelve discs, has to do with the feelings of guilt, shame, self-reproach, jealously, and/or suspicion.

Low back or lumbar pain is a reflection of the stored emotion of grief. This might explain the prevalence of low back pain in today's society. At least 80 percent of people have experienced or will experience low back pain in their lifetime. Think of all the unresolved grieving we go through; grieving over lost love, non-resonant relationships, death of a family member, friend, relative or pet. The unresolved

---

16 Singh, Narayan, *Messages from the Body*. Self-published, 1997.

emotions store up and finally are expressed as physical symptoms.

Sacral pain indicates fear, fear of current, past or future happenings.

From a chiropractic anatomical perspective, back pain can come from numerous sources. The surrounding and supportive spinal musculature may have been affected from poor posture, repetitive injury, poor lifting technique or trauma.

A 55-year-old woman presented at the clinic with neck and upper back pain. Her job is to assess computer chips using a microscope. She does this 8 to12 hours a day. Due to this posture she is reversing the natural c-shaped curve of her neck and putting stress on the supporting ligaments, discs and muscles. X-rays revealed not only reversal of spinal curvature, but also degenerative changes to the fifth disc of the neck.

She had been told by another health professional that this degeneration was only a sign of aging. I pointed out to her that the other discs, which looked full and healthy in her neck, were the same age as the one that was starting to break down. If it were age related then we should see similarities within all vertebra and discs of her spine. Her particular breakdown was not a sign of aging at all; only an indication of what she had been doing with her years as opposed to what the years had done to her.

Years of improper cervical spine curve, with the positioning at the microscope such that most of the stress was given at the lowest few vertebrae of the neck, caused them to break down faster. Thus degenerative changes in her vertebrae and discs resulted.

I once had the chance to compare the x-rays of a 75-year-old woman who had regular chiropractic care since childhood to the x-rays of a 35-year-old man, whose hobby was bronco-busting at rodeos. Although there are a multitude of factors involved with each person's life and health status, if you did not know the history or either person, you would think that the x-rays had been reversed. The woman had nice disc spaces with evenly contoured vertebral edges, and the man had advanced degenerative changes of his spine and discs.

Prolonged or repetitive postures create subluxations and have a way of slowly but steadily breaking down the tissues, regardless of the fact that you may have no pain.

When the pain shows up, the problem has been present sub-clinically for a long time, or lurking under the threshold of attention. It is only when the body is no longer able to adequately compensate for the subluxation that the pain begins.

The shock absorbers in the spine, the discs, can be injured through a number of means. Poor postures, improper lifting technique, torsional/twisting strain, or lifting things that are too heavy can all create strain on the discs and damage can occur. When discs become damaged, arm or leg referral of pain may happen also. You do not even need disc problems to experience headaches, jaw pain, arm or leg pain. Irritation on the nerve, the result of malposition of the vertebrae, and the irritation of the joints of the spine, is usually enough to cause these problems.

Evidence also suggests that someone who smokes is more predisposed to spinal pain than others. This is due to the adhering effects that nicotine has on the cells in the blood, resulting in less than effective nutrition to the spine and other parts of the body. Thus, faster breakdown of the body tissues and discs leading to decreased healing ability would occur.

From my perspective, correlating the patient's health complaint with muscle group involvement, organ dysfunction and emotional complexity helps me to diagnose the situation, discover meaning, and heal much more than just a "sore back."

For each pain there is a reason in the depths of the consciousness.

– Reinhold Voll

BACK TO YOU – THE JOURNEY CONTINUES

I have ceased to question stars and books; I have begun to listen to the teachings my blood whispers to me.

– Hermann Hesse[17]

The approach that I have taken in this chapter is one that allows an assessment of the function, biomechanics and physiology of the spine and nervous system. These serve as vehicles to enter into discussions with patients about their conditions or

17 Hesse, Hermann, as quoted in Levoy, ibid.

illnesses. It is through this that there is an opportunity to discuss the many ways to approach their health. People need direction to help them solve their own truths, hidden within their own body of knowledge. The chiropractic adjustment has a way of unlocking some of their truth and returning them toward health.

It is the patient practitioner, the observing practitioner, who by listening and acting with the heart and then speaking directly from the heart, who will have the patients with the most interesting of successes.

Homeopaths talk of an inner wisdom and provide remedies to not only alleviate conditions and symptoms but also cure the body by awakening that inner wisdom. Craniosacral therapists work with the inner physician. Chiropractors work with the Universal Intelligence or Innate of our body to help heal and improve immune function. I find that these are all paths to the same pinnacle. It is the body of knowledge that has the answers for us. It gives signals and guidance to help us discover our own healing path.

What I have found in clinical practice is that it is the deeper, underlying issues experienced throughout our lives, expressed outwardly as physical symptoms, which are the intangibles, the non-material, and thus not measurable. As such, there is no scientific rationale that can detect such intricacies nor explain these experiences. They just are.

We chiropractors work with the subtle substance of the soul. We release the imprisoned impulse, a tiny rivulet of force, that emanates from the mind and flows over the nerves to the cells and stirs them to life. We deal with the magic power that transforms common food into living, loving, thinking clay; that robes the earth with beauty, and hues and scents the flowers with the glory of the air....

– B.J.Palmer

Acknowledgements

I am grateful to my family and friends who contributed with love to this project.

Thank you to all my patients who continue to teach me each and every day.

– James Emmett

Conclusion

Where Do We Go From Here?

By Rudi Verspoor, FHCH, HD(RHom) DMH

Dean, Hahnemann College for Heilkunst
Director, Hahnemann Center for Heilkunst
Trustee, Hahnemann Center for Heilkunst Trust

WHERE DO WE GO FROM HERE?

Each person who enters the natural healing arts has undertaken his or her own journey of self-discovery. It is, despite the current growing popularity of the natural healing approach and alternatives to conventional medical practice, a path still less travelled for practitioners. To set out along a path that is not that marked by external authority but by an inner urging of the heart and conscience requires one to continually overcome fear and doubt and to have a commitment to truth over acceptance, monetary gain or status. Each such seeker of the truth within must be willing to become again like a child in order to learn new approaches, accept new insights and then integrate them into the older world-view. And yet, if we are to attain a true medical science grounded firmly in nature there must be pioneers who seek the unexplained.

This book is the story of several of these pioneering journeys by practitioners who started out with a more traditional approach and then found themselves searching for something that lay beyond the conventional. This search has taken them to looking beyond the outer appearances of illness to the inner meaning of symptoms and pain. In undertaking this journey, each practitioner has gained a deeper appreciation of the journey that each of their patients are on, and where on their path to healing they might be found.

We, as practitioners, cannot help our patients in terms of their inner development much beyond where we ourselves have gone. The deeper approach to the removal of disease and imbalance to allow for the restoration of health at all levels – body, mind, soul and spirit – demands a capacity for discernment that can only have come from the inner journey of the practitioner. In a sense, we are all, patient and practitioner, travelers along the road to soundness and wellness. It is our patients who become our teachers and encourage us to go further in our own inner journey and understanding of disease and remediation. To those who have, more is given. Where we open our hearts and minds to see and hear differently, we receive so much more and are then able to also give so much more.

More people today are looking for help along what they sense is a profound and singular journey to the self, even if they are uncertain as to how to do this or even what it fully means, much as the hero, Neo, in the movie The Matrix. They sense that health is more than the absence of symptoms, even if their conscious desire is to rid themselves of their pain and discomfort. They do not want a health specialist simply to tell them what to do in isolation from the other aspects of their existence, but to be a knowledgeable guide for them along the way to health, a way that can sometimes seem long and forbidding.

People are also looking for their practitioner to be part of a team that works harmoniously toward the same end – the health of the patient, but health in its broadest, highest and deepest sense, involving not just the body and intellect, but as much, if not more, the inner mind as well as the soul and spirit. If you are reading this book, you are one of these persons.

And yet, the path to wellness and soundness is strewn with confusion. Where to start and how to proceed in the world of natural health is by no means clear. The natural health field has grown enormously in the past decades, but it still lacks a coherent framework for the integration along rational principles of the myriad of therapies and approaches out there. Let's imagine an ideal clinic with a practitioner for each one of the more than 300 different therapies known, not to mention conventional medical options. You arrive and ask the receptionist where to go. You are handed a list of practitioners and therapies and told to pick one. There is currently no consistent or rational basis to tell you when you arrive where you should start and who you should go to see next. The onus lies on the patient to choose. Much of each person's treatment then becomes a matter of circumstances or unconscious choice. It can appear fortuitous or disheartening depending on the choices made.

What is needed is a system of medicine that encompasses the best of what different therapeutic approaches have to offer, both alternative and conventional and that is able to provide a clear jurisdiction for each therapy.

Currently, there is no common means of identifying a disease or imbalance. The dominant approach usually mistakes the effect or result for the cause. The actual cause remains hidden and medicine too often descends into the management of symptoms (usually by suppressive, and often toxic means, because to be able to cure means to be able to identify the true cause). Thus, we have labels such as asthma, chronic fatigue, arthritis, and allergies, all of which hide the reason for these conditions. To name an effect or manifestation of disease as the disease is thereby to draw a veil over the cause so that the practitioner is forced to look through a glass darkly. The real question must always be, what has caused this set of symptoms, this pain or discomfort. However, the search for the cause is all too often undertaken in the wrong place because of certain prejudices or preconceptions.

The conventional model effectively sees disease as a material thing, and therefore the cause is to be sought only on the material plane, in the realm of the physical, material body and bio-chemistry. The reductionist nature of modern material science has done wonders in terms of its ability to read what is happening at the physical level, but it has blinded itself from looking beyond the outer appearances into the deeper aspects of man's being.

While we know privately that man is as much a soul and spirit as a collection of bio-chemical elements, the current paradigm demands effectively that the patient leave his soul and spirit at the door of the consulting room, for it is not officially recognized by the allopathic medical model. We know that the heart is not simply a pump, but the carrier of many soul qualities and that people can literally die of a "broken heart." However, there is nothing in what is taught conventionally that validates this private knowing. In essence, both practitioner and patient must accept a form of schizophrenia when trying to heal – looking at the obvious and ignoring the deeper, underlying causation of disease.

There is a famous story of a wise man who was renowned for his wisdom, but was also a little absent-minded. One evening, some friends came across him on his knees under the streetlight searching for something. When asked, he stated that he was looking for his glasses. Wanting to help, they queried where he had lost his glasses, so they could render their help most effective. The wise man told them he had lost his glasses behind the house. Astonished, his friends asked him why he was here in front of the house looking for his lost glasses instead of at the back. The wise man told them, "Because the light is better here."

All too often we look where the light has been provided by our training rather than in the darker recesses of the mind and soul, where the truth often lies, particularly the truth about wholeness. What is needed is a science of these deeper recesses of our being as much as we have a science for its physical, bio-chemical aspects.

Heilkunst provides the rational framework to develop this direction. To do this requires the cooperation of practitioners in each field, each with a comprehension of the context of disease and treatment, and each understanding what their particular therapy or discipline brings that is unique and when that should be used in a given case. The practitioners in this book have all undertaken to study Heilkunst and to begin the difficult, yet rewarding process of creating an integrated system of treatment that addresses the whole person yet is firmly grounded in natural law principle, respecting the jurisdiction of each therapy. It is not a question as to whether a given therapy can remove asthma, for example, as each can furnish examples of such successful cases, but rather a question as to which case of asthma will be cured by which therapy.

Asthma, as a condition, or result of disease or imbalance, has many causes, and each case will be different. The label asthma becomes meaningless as a guide to the cause. If it is due to a misaligned spine, then spinal manipulation will help; if it is due to emotional traumas in childhood that are not too deeply embedded in the somatic realm yet, then psychotherapy will help. The one cannot work where the cause does not fall within its jurisdiction. The science of health is to determine the exact scope of each therapy: under what circumstances and for what causes is it valid?

While all therapies can have an effect in relieving pain in many cases, the objective of a rational system of medicine is to remove the cause. Only when a therapy acts within its jurisdiction does it achieve that, instead of simply relief or palliation. It is the task of Heilkunst to establish these jurisdictions, and to offer this rational system to the patient so that they might be truly freed from their pain and suffering, not by suppressing the symptoms, but by removing the cause(s) according to natural law. If we work against nature, we may obtain temporary relief, but we must also sacrifice a certain degree of our life force and our being in the process. We become less whole, not more.

As the founder of Heilkunst stated in the very first paragraph of his book setting out the framework of a true system of remediation, "The physician's highest and only calling is to make the sick healthy, to cure, as it is called." To do so, there must be a system of treatment that is based on "clearly realizable principles."

The practitioners in this book have opened their minds to this end and their stories testify to their commitment to find the truth so that their patients may receive the benefit. With their help and with the help of many others, we will be able to advance the science of medicine into the deeper realms of human existence and be able to restore health with true causal prescribing.

– Rudi Verspoor, FHCH, HD(RHom) DMH

OPEN MINDS

A New Perspective on Healing

Copies of this book may be ordered from:

Rudi Verspoor
The Hahnemann College for Heilkunst
2411 River Road, Ottawa ON, K4M 1B4
Telephone: 613-830-8307

Dr. Farid Shodjaee
St. Laurent Dental Centre, Ottawa, ON
Telephone: 613-744-6611, ext. 241
E-mail: farid@drfarid.com

Mary Rothschild
Telephone: 613-692-6464
E-mail: natrldoc@rogers.com

Dr. James Emmett
Centrum Chiropractic and Acupuncture Clinic,
Ottawa, ON
Telephone: 613-830-4080
E-mail: DrEmmett@bellnet.ca